GW00792330

Leprosy and a
Life in South India

Leprosy and a Life in South India

Journeys with a Tamil Brahmin

James Staples

LEXINGTON BOOKS
Lanham • Boulder • New York • Toronto • Plymouth, UK

Published by Lexington Books
A wholly owned subsidiary of Rowman & Littlefield
4501 Forbes Boulevard, Suite 200, Lanham, Maryland 20706
www.rowman.com

10 Thornbury Road, Plymouth PL6 7PP, United Kingdom

Copyright © 2014 by Lexington Books

All rights reserved. No part of this book may be reproduced in any form or by any electronic or mechanical means, including information storage and retrieval systems, without written permission from the publisher, except by a reviewer who may quote passages in a review.

British Library Cataloguing in Publication Information Available

Library of Congress Cataloging-in-Publication Data

ISBN: 978-0-7391-8734-0 (cloth: alk paper)
ISBN: 978-0-7391-8735-7 (electronic)

∞™ The paper used in this publication meets the minimum requirements of American National Standard for Information Sciences Permanence of Paper for Printed Library Materials, ANSI/NISO Z39.48-1992.

Printed in the United States of America

For Felix, Theo, Immanuel and Bhavani

Contents

Acknowledgments

This book has been a long time in the making and, as always with these kinds of projects, I have accrued many debts along the way. My greatest thanks, of course, go to Das himself, as well as to the cast of his friends, acquaintances and family who also gave up their time to talk to me about him, and those in Anandapuram who continued to receive me so hospitably on my frequent return trips. Particular thanks are due to Gopal Rao, Venkata Subbaiah, Mamalla and Kanakadurga.

The UK's Association of Social Anthropologists' (ASA) conference on "The Interview" in 2010, organized by Jonathan Skinner in Belfast, provided me with the ideal opportunity to discuss (and refine) some of the ideas that underpinned my project. I am grateful to my fellow panellists, Pat Caplan, Judith Okely and Isak Niehaus for their comments and insights, as well as additional feedback from Katherine Smith and Nigel Rapport (with whom I subsequently edited a book on biography and the ethnographic interview), as well as from Kristine Harris, who commented helpfully on a draft of the paper I presented at the conference. Jacky Bonney, in Delhi, generously read chapters for me as I produced them and commented via email along the way, while Tom Widger and Becky Sutherland offered feedback on the completed draft. Becky, in addition, put up with being a sounding board for sentences and paragraphs as I wrote them, and with my prolonged retreats to my writing shed in the garden. The demands of our sons Theo and Felix offered welcome relief on my return to the house each evening.

It was through discussions with my colleagues Andrew Beatty and Isak Niehaus at Brunel – both of whom were engaged at the time in their own experiments with ethnographic writing—that I developed the confidence to adopt the format for telling Das's story that I have (although it goes without saying that its failings remain my own). The final product has been further shaped by the gentle but incisive direction of Amy King, Associate Editor at Lexington Books, and her assistant Kelly Blackburn (as well as their anonymous readers). I am hugely grateful to them for their faith, patience, guidance and clarity throughout the process, making the final editing of the manuscript a genuine pleasure.

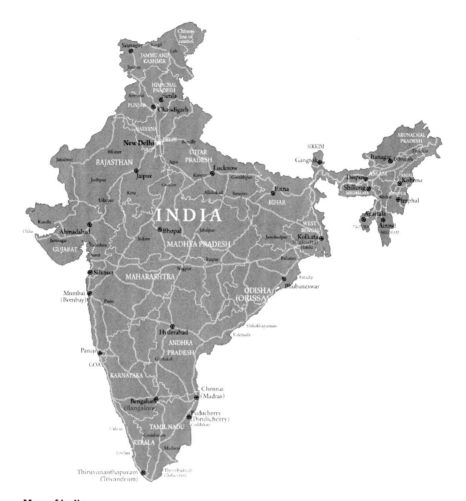

Map of India

Prologue

The first time I saw him he was still G. Mohandas Iyer.[1] The "G" stood in for his father's given name, Gajavakra, a name derived from the elephant-headed Hindu God, Ganesh. Literally, it translated as Ganesh's twisted trunk, a symbol of knowledge and spiritual progress.[2] "Mohandas" was the name bestowed upon him by his parents—one shared with the Mahatma himself, suggesting they were supporters of the Indian National Congress party. The 'Iyer' surname reinforced the likelihood: it marked him out as a particular kind of Tamil Brahmin, a member of one of the ritually highest caste group-ings in the state who, in the early years after independence, dominated the political arena. A name, in South India, could tell you a lot, although prob-ably not as much as it hid.

A week later, by which time I had left India to return to England, Mohan-das had become someone else. He had undergone a Christian baptism; had married a girl twenty-years his junior who came from what many still saw as an untouchable caste; and had taken over the corner of a desk I had been occupying for the past six months in a leprosy colony's administrative office. He also had a new name: Tejagani Jobdas. Whereas in Tamil Nadu, his native state, it was usual to take your father's given name in place of a family name—hence the "G" that had prefixed his Mohandas—where he now lived in Andhra Pradesh, the next state up on India's eastern coastline, names were done differently. Here, family names passed, unaltered, down through the male line, much like an English surname, except that they were then abbrevi-ated to the initial letter and placed in front of the given name.

When Mohandas's father Gajavakra had shifted, several years earlier, from Tamil Nadu to Andhra and, as a poor man, had registered for a ration card to use at the Government's subsidized rice stores, he was asked for his family name. Gajavakra gave the name of his own father, Tejaswami. The official, who had not heard properly but who was not bothered enough to ask Gajavakra to repeat it, wrote down "Tejagani." The name stuck.

When Mohandas finally came to live with his father in Andhra many years later, he too adopted Tejagani as his house name. Jobdas, his new Christian name, was the one that had come into the pastor's head as he baptised him: a name derived from the Old Testament's *Book of Job*, describing a patient man tested by God. "What does it matter?" Jobdas said to me when I asked him, years later, whether he minded his name being changed by the sleight of a bureaucrat's hand and the whim of a pastor he had only just met. "It's only a name." There were far more pressing things to worry about. And if the two cities where he spent his most formative years, Madras and Bombay, could also change their names—to Chennai and Mumbai, respectively—why couldn't he?

The next time I encountered Jobdas, eighteen months later, was at Bombay International Airport, 750 miles west, on the opposite coastline. Charging toward the exit with my luggage trolley, wilfully ignoring the multiple offers to take my bags, provide me with a taxi, a rickshaw or a cheap hotel room, I also ignored the man in the bright blue shirt who put out his arm and called, "Sir! Sir!" But, as I passed him, I realized he was calling my name: "James, James sir! Please, it's Mr. Jobdas, sir!"

That I had failed to recognize him was not surprising. The last and only time I had seen him was through the bamboo struts that held the conical leaf roof above the low mud walls of the circular office building in which I had been working. On that occasion, Jobdas's father—the man once called Gajavakra but, since his own conversion, renamed Timothy—had left Jobdas there while he came inside. He had entered in the hope of finding his son, with whom he had recently been reunited after spending more than a decade apart, some work. Jobdas was nearly thirty-five years old, had completed his secondary education, could write well in English and was skilled with numbers, Timothy told the woman in charge of the office, Emma (or Sister Cox, as she was more formally known: foreigners had multiple names too, with similarly complex histories). He could also speak Tamil, Hindi and Marathi fluently, and was working on his Telugu, the local language. Give him a job, Timothy had pleaded, and his son would marry the girl they had found and stay with him and his own wife in the village; without one, he would wander here and there (as, it much later transpired, had often been his want) with nothing to do and no means of supporting himself.

I cannot remember now, nearly three decades on, the ins and the outs of Timothy's conversation with Emma Cox that morning. I was leaving the next day and my mind was on other things. But I do know that luck was on Jobdas's side. Solly, the English man who had, for several years, kept the accounts in that office—serenely cross-legged on the floor, immaculate in white handloom pyjams and collarless shirt, sandwiched between two metal trunks full of ledgers—had not returned from his last retreat to an ashram several months earlier. There was work that needed to be done, and it was Jobdas—or Das, to which I shall abbreviate him—who would end up doing it.

Emma had told me about him in her letters, but that day at the airport back in August 1986—where she had sent him to meet me—was our first proper meeting. We travelled back into central Bombay on one of the decrepit state buses and, after walking for a while in the direction of Victoria Terminus, he finally turned off and marched us down some stairs to an air-conditioned coffee shop he had found earlier. Without consulting either the menu, or me, he ordered us South Indian coffees, which were brought to the table in mottled-brown china cups. Das was thinner then, and his thick hair, carefully sculpted with coconut oil, was still naturally black. But he exuded the same nervous energy that continued to characterise his bodily movements more than two decades later: fingers strumming impatiently on the table during our conversation, neatly trimmed moustache twitching, and eyes flitting quickly from side-to-side, always alert to what might be going on around him. We spent maybe an hour there, in the dark coolness of that coffee shop, *Abba* playing disconcertingly on the music system in the background, catching up on news of people we both knew and establishing shared ground. I had returned for a second six-month stint as a volunteer at the leprosy colony, Anandapuram, where Das now lived and worked. Emma Cox, the colony's administrator, was the aunt of one of my school friends, and it was through that connection that I had come to be there in the first place: a school leaver, taking what was meant to be a single year off before going to University, volunteering for a small NGO. I had taught English classes, helped set up a rudimentary printing press, and carried out routine correspondence.

Emerging from the café back into the intense stickiness of the street and the brightness of the mid-morning sun, it took me a few moments to regain my bearings. Even with Das carrying my heaviest bag, I struggled to keep up as he dodged through the traffic to cross the road to the station, where— eventually—we reached the waiting room. "Here," he said, pointing to a long, unoccupied wooden bench. "Put your bags underneath, and you can lie down and take some rest."

"Aren't we going to stay in the Red Shield?" I was referring to the Salvation Army's well-known guest house in Colaba where I had stayed on previous visits to Bombay. It was cool again here, beneath the ceiling fan— and probably more salubrious than the dormitories of the guest house—but it was also noisier and busier than anywhere I would usually envisage taking a rest, and there was nowhere to leave my luggage unattended.

"No need for that," Das replied, breezily. "I'm going to arrange us reservations so we can travel back tonight itself. No need to waste your money on accommodation unnecessarily. And you can rest here while I get everything organized!"

With that, he was off, only returning six hours later to take me for something to eat and then down to the platform to board our train. "Where have you been all this time?" I asked. I was exasperated at having been left stranded for so long, but too pleased to see him back to make much fuss. Excited at being in India again, I had not been interested in sleeping, and after the first couple of hours of reading and watching the Bombay world go past from my hard wooden bench I had grown increasingly restless.

"Just sorting things out," he said, cryptically. I never found out where he had been for sure, and he claims to have forgotten, but—knowing what I now know—I could make some reasonable guesses.

Finding answers to the questions I built up in relation to Das over the next quarter of a century is one of the reasons I wanted to carry out the research for this book. There were so many loose threads, so many gaps, so many contradictions that I could not account for in the scraps of narrative I heard or picked up—out of order, as and when, in all kinds of different contexts—that I felt compelled to fill at least some of them in. Listening to people's narrative accounts of their lives, as I discovered in the process, was a very good way of documenting the politics of representation, with the act of telling such stories also serving as part of a project of identity formation.[3]

Had his stories been mundane, perhaps I would not have bothered. But Das's life, for the most part, had not been mundane. After reading *Q & A*, the Vikas Swarup novel on which the subsequent film *Slumdog millionaire* was based, Das often compared his life self-consciously to that of the Ram Mohammad Thomas, the main protagonist.[4] He had not yet reached the happy ending imagined in the book, but he had, he said, encountered similar scrapes along the way.

Born a Brahmin in a rural backwater of southern Tamil Nadu, Das had ended up living, for several years, on the streets of both Bombay and Madras, surviving as an unofficial station porter, hotel tout and sometime tourist guide. He had won and lost fortunes on horse races, bets on infamous numbers rackets, and on running card schools. He knew, at first hand, the pleasures to be had in Bombay's red light district, and—in a nation sometimes described as deeply conservative—had enjoyed a number of sexual encounters and illicit relationships. But for all the fun and the freedom that he described, he had also encountered violence and hardship, including time in police cells and prisons in both Bombay and Madras, before the dramatic reunions with family members that once again shifted his life trajectory.

It was not the kind of life one might associate with a Tamil Brahmin called G. Mohandas Iyer. The short hand explanation for his diversion from a likelier path was that, at nineteen, he was also diagnosed with leprosy: a disease that is curable and which never killed anyone, but which became a near universal symbol of stigma and social death. Such was the power of leprosy's connotations that, in the popular imagination, in one swoop it rendered even the highest Hindu castes untouchable and unemployable.[5] Leprosy played a major role in how Das's life panned out. He would not, to be sure, have spent the best part of thirty years living in a leprosy colony without it. But, as it started to become clear as we explored his life story, leprosy was only one of several competing factors that shaped what happened to him from the late 1960s onwards. Leprosy and people's reactions to it, I discovered, shoulder the blame for a whole range of social ills and provide cover for still more uncomfortable realities.[6] Officials were not adverse to such explanations either: if the ill treatment of those with leprosy could be blamed on the superstitions of the uneducated, it served as a useful mask for the structural poverty and deprivation that also contributed to patients' hardships.[7]

A full biographical account—a "warts and all" picture, as Das liked to describe it—has the power to challenge the conventional wisdom on leprosy, and to illustrate graphically that people's identities are multiple, complex and ever changing. It also, apart from offering a good story, has the potential to say something more generalisable about a life and a time: something about what it was like to grow up in mid-century India, come of age in the 1960s, and live against the backdrop of all the political and social upheavals that shaped the decades which followed.[8] That was the other reason I wanted to write Das's story. As an anthropologist—a profession I took up as a direct response to my experiences in India in the 1980s—I had spent a lot of time reading about and researching the structures that are said to underpin Indian life: things like Hinduism, the caste system, ritual purity and pollution, marriage and the extended family. Whether or not these things as they are practiced or understood in the present were intrinsically Indian, products of a prolonged encounter with colonial rule or figments of scholars' imaginations is, in a sense, beside the point: they are categories that continue to inform discussion and experience of India, even alongside new foci on modernity, diasporas and globalisation. To the people I worked with, these things still mattered, but not necessarily in the structured ways we might imagine.

When newspapers, magazines and travel books beyond India concern themselves with these issues, they tend to conceive of them as fixed: as "the ancient caste system"—set against western notions of egalitarianism—or as the "rules of Hindu belief." They offer a static lens that is woefully inadequate for capturing the dynamism of Indian life. Conventional ethnographies and scholarly papers offer, as one might expect, far more nuanced analyses, but the level of abstraction required to draw out wider theoretical insights often render our texts far from anything our informants would recognize as descriptions of their lives. Looked at through the prism of an individual life, however, abstract categories like caste or religion morph into something else altogether. Caste, for Das, is not so much a constraining structure that ranks him alongside others, but more a quality that shapes his whole identity and his perspective on the world. It changes the way he moves, what he eats, what he does, how he sees others and how they see him.[9] Having leprosy, and even marrying someone from a caste he perceived to be right at the other end of the spectrum does not negate, from his perspective, his essential Brahmin-ness, even as his perception of what it is to be a Brahmin shifts across time. It continues to inform everything he does. Likewise, despite his conversion to Christianity, tracing Das's life story also taught me something about how particular Hindu ideas are lived: not as abstract, intellectual notions, but as embodied dispositions.[10] Following Das's narrative across time, and reading over and again the transcripts of what I had at first heard only as throw away remarks, demonstrated that fact to me in ways that, I think, conventional participant observation would have been hard pressed to reveal.

Das's story, then, offers a snapshot of life in South India through one man's eyes—constrained, but not over-determined by, gender, caste and class—at particular points in its recent history: from a village in the Kaveri delta in Tamil Nadu in 1950, just after Indian independence, to Madras (now Chennai), Bombay (now Mumbai) and Hyderabad, as well as many years in a leprosy colony. In addition to receiving treatment there for his own disease, he was also, for a time, in charge. "I've had an up-and-down life," he once told me, as we travelled to one of the places he had lived by train. "I was born a Brahmin, but ended up living on the streets, all on my own. And from there I came to run a leprosy colony, with a wife and children, and ended up, again, with more or less nothing!" But although his is a deeply personal account, a life like no other, it also remains one that tells more generalisable truths. Arnold and Blackburn, in introducing the contributions that make up their influential volume, *Telling Lives in India,* sum up the value of life histories very succinctly:

> [L]ife histories should not be seen as . . . a narrowing down or even a disavowal of grand themes . . . Rather, life histories enable us to render more intelligible precisely the complex of forces at work in modern societies and to reflect further, and from more solid foundations, on many of the major themes that dominate the subcontinent—gender, modernity, colonialism and nationalism, religion, social changes, family and kinship, and interrelationship between self and society.[11]

In Das's case, the themes to which his stories speak might even extend beyond India. On one of our train journeys between the places where he had lived, for example, Das dipped into my copy of *Venus on Wheels* by Gelya Frank, an anthropologist's biographical account of an American woman called Diane DeVries, born without arms or legs.[12] It had been part of my background reading as I grappled to find appropriate ways of dealing with the material I was accumulating. Das, by contrast, was reading it to kill time between Chennai and Mumbai after finishing his Tamil detective novel, but he soon became engrossed. "Her life reads just like mine!" he said. When I expressed surprise that he, as an Indian Brahmin man who had been affected by leprosy, should find much in common with a white, working class suburban American woman born without limbs, he explained that DeVries, too, had had an "up-and-down sort of life," in which things did not just get progressively better or worse in a linear trajectory, but shifted back and forth in a much messier, less narratively convenient, fashion across time.

A final reason for writing this book—or at least for doing the research on which it draws—is that I wanted to explore the relationship between the anthropologist and his or her research assistants: those local people who, although sometimes even credited in the by-lines of our books, somehow remain in the background. Das, as well as becoming a close friend over the years, also worked for me—for more than two years, in total—as a paid research assistant, and was a major informant for several more. He was central to the research, affecting the way I came to see and understand the lives I encountered in the field, but in my academic writings his contributions are only made manifest at occasional junctures along the way—a pithy quote, maybe, or an anonymized anecdote to illustrate a point. Like other informants, he serves as a social commentator and, sometimes, an analyst of the social realities he observes. But what remain hidden are the fights, the shared experiences and the in-jokes that make the sharing of those insights a possibility in the first place. Research assistants are not simply conduits of data; they actively partake in the construction of that data.[13] This book is a tribute to Das's role, for better and for worse, in the research process. Reliving some of our disagreements—performed as they were against the sultry backdrop of South Indian cityscapes—was not always comfortable. Neither of us comes out particularly well in the documenting of them. But it is potentially useful, we agreed, to unpick what is, we expect, a fairly typical relationship in the creation of anthropological material.

For readers keen to get to the story, it begins, back in 1950, at the start of the next chapter. In what is left of this one, however, I want to say something about how we did the research for this book[14] and how I wrote it, as well as to locate the text within a wider anthropological genre and to consider the ethical implications of embarking on such a project.

Methodologically, the book draws on my own, first hand knowledge of Das's life and my records of it, strewn throughout my more general field notes, and, more particularly, on a long series of taped interviews and conversations over the summers of 2009 and 2011. I also interviewed and talked to some of those close to him. Back in 2000, along with others in Anandapuram, Das kept, at my request, an informant diary and, when we were working together in Hyderabad from mid-2005 until the end of 2006, a separate set of field notes so that I could compare our perspectives on events. Since 1990, I have also been a trustee of a small UK charity that raises funds for some of the work going on in Anandapuram and, in this capacity, worked on a newsletter, produced two or three times a year, for supporters of the charity. Although the material presented there is highly edited, much of it draws on letters Das wrote to me at the time, and was—at the very least—useful for cross-checking dates and the chronology of Das's later account (which was, I discovered, remarkably accurate).

In terms of our most recent interviews, Das and I usually spoke in the early mornings, either side of breakfast, or in the evenings, after dinner, on the verandah of what had once been Emma Cox's house, and part of which now served as an occasional kitchen for guests to the community. It was a relatively neutral, shaded place on the outskirts of the village, and while we were disturbed often, we attracted less attention than if we had spoken at, say, Das's own house, where neighbours would have congregated together very quickly.

We also travelled back to some of the places that featured in Das's earlier narratives: to his ancestral home in Tamil Nadu, where I saw the place where he was born and where the village headman showed us around and entertained us with South Indian coffee; to Kumbakonam and Chennai and the various locations where he and his family had lived and where his father had opened up canteens and fast-food stands; to the station platforms where he spent more than a decade working as an unofficial porter, hotel tout and sometime tourist guide; and to the race courses where he had won and lost his fortunes. In several of these locations, and especially on the station platforms, we ran into people who had known and lived with Das and who had featured in the accounts he had given during our taped interviews. It was this literal reconstruction of Das's movements—by going back to the places where he had spent formative time and which he considered important in his life trajectory, by walking through them and, to borrow Ingold's phrase, taking a "dwelling perspective" [15] —that was innovative about this particular approach to recording life stories. Our journeys gave shape and colour to his stories. The events and places he described suddenly came to life and made sense in ways they previously had not. For Das, going back also transformed the ways in which he resurrected the memories he had been drawing upon. Elements of the story that appeared missing from earlier accounts were forthcoming on location, as were anecdotes about people not previously mentioned.

This approach was inspired, initially, by my reading, several years earlier, of Michel de Certeau's short essay 'Walking in the City,'[16] a piece that recognizes how our movements through spaces, never wholly determined by the overarching visions of city planners and architects, in themselves shape the social worlds in which we live. As Ingold and Vergunst put it a few years later, "social relations . . . are not enacted *in situ* but are paced out along the ground";[17] literally, in the cases they and their contributors describe, by walking. The insights I drew from this served as inspirational sparks rather than as directives, but they certainly heightened my consciousness of the fact that movements were no less important in the meaningful re-telling of Das's life than the words that came out of his mouth. For us, as we shifted across India, retracing his steps, many of our movements were on trains and buses, or huddled together into auto- and cycle rickshaws, rather than on foot. But it was still through these movements—and the sounds, sights and smells that accompanied them—that places were woven together and the telling of Das's stories became possible.

This is not, of course, to say that the newer, richer versions of his stories were necessarily more objectively accurate than the synoptic accounts of the past. He was still involved in editing and representing his life in certain ways and to particular effect, often self-consciously framing his life as being, in his words, "just like a cinema film." Das was a keen viewer of popular Tamil, Telugu and Hindi movies, as well as being an avid reader of Tamil detective novellas. Exposure to these and other genres of story telling clearly shaped the form that his stories took, offering him templates through which to construct his own account. It was certainly a different kind of narrative to those I collected from less literate informants, or from those less accustomed to my particular ways of working. Nevertheless, for all his presentational techniques, our most recent interviews were much richer than earlier accounts, and less self-consciously about the overall impression his stories might create when edited back together.

My case for conducting the interviews in the scattered ways that I did is perhaps comparable to the case Jeanette Marie Mageo makes for using figurative dream analysis in ethnographic fieldwork.[18] When we ask people questions, as she explains it, they are often reticent about disclosing feelings and behaviours that diverge from the norms they have internalized. In dreams, however, because these divergent feelings are encrypted in symbols, description of their content might allow people to disclose that to which they have not even admitted to themselves. Das was not, of course, inadvertently revealing a more candid version of the events that had shaped his life through descriptions of his dreams; he was, most of the time, all too aware that he was speaking on the record. However, in telling his stories over time, out of chronological order and in different contexts, they became less anchored in the over-arching narrative structure that Das gave to the story of his life in shorter accounts. In focusing in on the parts he surrendered some of the control he might otherwise have had over how the whole came to be represented. This made our later interviews, at least from my perspective, more richly informative.

In the past, when I had asked Das to tell me his story, he had summarized it in less than an hour. It was always a tale of a positive beginning wrecked by the onset of leprosy, closely followed by his remarkable ascent from vagrant station porter to chief functionary of an NGO. This was useful in telling me what was important to him—or at least what he thought was important that I should know about—but it clearly skipped over key events in order to focus on what he saw as central themes. It also ended in around 1995, before things went awry again and the positive ending that rounded off the story so well was spoiled. I needed ways of getting beyond the obvious.

Beyond interviews "on location," then, my subsequent approach was to use his standard narrative as an entry point to particular events and to get him to elaborate upon them, interjecting with subsidiary questions and prompts along the way. After each interview I would transcribe the recordings and read them through, drawing out further, more probing questions each time, and returning to points that I did not understand or if I was confused about chronology. In this way, the interviews became more and more detailed— and covered shorter and shorter periods of history—each time. The result was between thirty and forty hours of recordings and a pile of notes, comple- mented with the secondary materials I described above.

Collecting the material was, in some ways, the easy part. I had, after all, known Das on and off for the best part of three decades and had a good rapport with him, and I had already lived through and recorded many of the key events of his story from different perspectives. More daunting was the prospect of what came next: the writing-up of his account in a way that not only spoke to wider themes and theories of interest to anthropologists of South Asia—if not more widely still—but which remained recognizable as *his* (or, at least, *our*) own story.

There is always, of course, a disjuncture between the visceral experience of ethnographic practice and the written texts we produce to represent those experiences. Indeed, one of the purposes of the anthropological endeavour is to draw out more generalizable insights and theories about social life from the particular, concrete events that we observe and participate in. At the same time, recognition of writing as an act of violence in and of itself has become a commonplace in the post "Writing Culture" era,[19] with the problems of authorship and power well documented and reflected upon. This is not the place to revisit in detail those debates, influential though they have been on how the chapters that follow take shape. What troubled me in particular, however, was what happened to people's stories—to the stuff of their every- day lives—when we synthesized them to illustrate or illuminate theoretical and thematic concerns that are only tangentially, if at all, related to the original contexts of those experiences. A vignette about village life might find its way into an academic conversation about, for example, agency versus structure, or about ontological commensurability cross-culturally. Ethnographic insights might well (and indeed *should*) inform and help shape those debates, but at the same time they can render the lives that informed them scarcely recognizable to those who were living them. Andrew Beatty, in making a case for what he calls "narrative ethnography," summarizes the problem very neatly: "The people in our case studies are in unwitting dialogue with the people in other ethnographies; they are never merely themselves." Writing-up becomes "a curious renunciation of the life around you"[20] rather than an affirmation of it. Joseph Alter faced similar difficulties in trying to impose order on what his long-time friend and informant, a low-caste Himalayan hunter and milk seller, told him. "My efforts at classification," he came to realize, "seemed to undermine precisely that which made him human."[21] Both authors make an important point: I know that even if I were to translate many of the articles I have written into Telugu, purge them of anthropological jargon and offer to read them out loud, most, if not all, of my informants—even if I could persuade them to listen—would have difficulty in making sense of what I had made of the experiences they shared with me. In working out how to tell Das's story, I had what I saw as an ethical commitment to present something that both he and those who know him would recognize. At the same time, by allowing readers to make connections with wider human concerns, I also wanted to make a contribution to the ethnographic record of South Asia as well as to a wider discussion about anthropological methods and styles of ethnographic writing.

The difficulty in pulling that off was not so much in the act of writing itself; adopting a relatively straightforward narrative form and allowing character, motivation and action to emerge gradually out of the stories rather than trying to extract those elements allowed the words to flow, perhaps unsurprisingly, more easily than they had during most of my other writing projects. I felt, for once, that I was writing with rather than against the grain. But it was not just that writing this way was easier. It also, it seemed to me, enabled the complexities of social practice to emerge much more clearly, contradictions intact, than in conventional ethnography, where case studies often need to be shoehorned to fit the arguments we want to make. As Chernoff points out, stories can actually be more revealing than what we learn from analyses based on abstract concepts.[22] This narrative style of writing also allowed the wider insights on South Asian social institutions that Das's stories brought out to emerge embedded in specific, historically contingent circumstances. We learn versions of what happened in the past and can begin to understand how it has shaped a particular kind of present.

It was for these reasons—that narrative accounts could potentially tell us more, or at least something else—that I found it important to resist earlier suggestions from my publisher to guard against making the text "*too* accessible." A style that appeared insufficiently academic, they feared, might lead scholars to think that the book was not for them. In making my case I was fortunate that there is a long tradition in anthropology, as well as several decades of experimental ethnographies, that I could point to. It was not until I had written-up the main body of Das's account and was scouting around for material that would help me reflect on it and place it in wider anthropological context, however, that I realized quite how long-established the life history genre within the discipline was. Such accounts, I discovered, can be traced— at least in American anthropology—as far back as the 1920s, to the same era in which Malinowski was establishing fieldwork-based ethnography as the discipline's standard.[23] The earliest examples appeared mostly to be accounts of the lives of native Americans, such as Paul Radin's *Crashing Thunder*,[24] the so-called autobiography of a Winnebago tribe member, Sam Blowsnake, in 1926, or Leo Simmons' *Sun Chief*[25] in 1942.[26] Mary Smith's *Baba of Karo*,[27] published in 1954, helped to extend the regional scope of the genre, emerging out of a friendship struck up between the author and a Muslim Hausa girl she met while conducting fieldwork in Nigeria.

Sidney Mintz references all of these books in what has become an anthropological classic of the genre: *Worker in the Cane: A Puerto Rican Life History*.[28] First published in 1960, Mintz's book differed from most of the earlier accounts, he claimed, because of its focus on a "westernized working class person"—a man called Taso who, with his "restless and inquiring mind" and well-developed capacity for reflection in some ways bears an uncanny resemblance to Das, my own protagonist. Perhaps our choices of subject say more about us as authors than we initially imagine. As Crapanzano notes in one of his own experiments with the genre—a 1980 life history account of an Arab Moroccan tile maker called Tuhami,[29] styled, as he puts it, to shock us from our complacency—our most popular biographical subjects are those with whom we share similarities as well as empathy and profound difference. Tuhami—like Das, or Mintz's interlocutor, Taso—identifies himself, like the anthropologist, as an outsider, ordinary in many ways and yet, at the same time, extraordinary. In several instances, too, the starting point for our inquiries is also one of bafflement in the face of an enigma. In Mintz's case, for example, Taro's sudden and apparently unexpected religious conversion was the catalyst for his investigation. For me, it was Das's unaccounted for disappearances from the village and the murkiness of his financial affairs that piqued my curiosity.

In all of these cases, friendship—for better and for worse—had a profound impact on the nature of the research undertaken.[30] Mintz reflects, for example, on how Taso held back from telling him about religious conversion at the time it happened not because he was a stranger but, on the contrary, because, as his friend, he feared his disapproval. Karen McCarthy Brown describes a comparable problem in her "intimate spiritual biography" of a

Vodou priestess living in Brooklyn, New York. "As Alourdes and I became friends," she writes in the introduction to her book, *Mama Lola*,[31] "I found it increasingly difficult to maintain an uncluttered image of myself as a scholar and researcher in her presence. This difficulty brought about a change in the research I was doing. As I got closer to Alourdes, I got closer to Vodou. The Vodou Alourdes practices is intimate and intense, and I soon found that I could not claim a place in her Vodou family and remain a detached observer."[32] While some might consider her subsequent initiation into Vodou a step too far, I am sympathetic to her claim that when the distinction between participant observer and informant breaks down, intellectual labour can be brought into closer relation with life as it is experienced by those we work with.[33] In short, she recognizes—as do the other authors I have cited—the limits of ethnography.

Within South Asia, there have also been several life history accounts. In common with the genre more generally, they tend to focus on those whose stories are usually left out from official discourse. James Freeman's *Untouchable*[34]—the first life history account I read, several years before working out how to present Das's story—is, as its name suggests, the story of a former untouchable, a man called Muli, from Orissa. It was finding the son of one of my informants, the literate sixteen-year-old son of leprosy-affected parents who later went on to university, engrossed in my copy the book that first convinced me it *was* possible to write scholarly material that could also appeal to a wider readership. *Knowing Dil Das*,[35] by Joseph Alter, likewise takes an untouchable—a Himalayan hunter and *dudwallah* (milk trader)—as its central character, as do Vasant Moon's autobiography *Growing Up Untouchable in India*[36] and Viramma's *Viramma: Life of An Indian Untouchable*.[37] The first two, while they quote their protagonists at length, are clearly biographies; the words of Muli and Dil Das interlaced with comment and analysis by their authors, the relationship between anthropologist and subject a central theme. Moon's book, on the other hand, although translated from his mother tongue Marathi into English by sociologist Gail Omvedt and preceded with an introduction from historian Eleanor Zelliot, is written entirely in the first person—the account of a highly literate civil servant. *Viramma* is also a translated first person account, and—beyond a very short contextualisation chapter at the very end and a glossary of terms—is presented entirely in her own voice (at least in the English translation). Unlike Moon, however, Viramma can neither read nor write, and her collaborators—Josiane and Jean-Luc Racine—clearly played a significant role in delivering Viramma's words, captured over a decade of interviews, on to the page.[38]

For all the differences between individual examples, this well-established life history genre, coupled with a post-1980s call for us to reflect on the role of the author and the politics of representation in all our texts, clearly had an impact—conscious and otherwise—on the kind of book I ended up writing.

But the immediate impetus to write it in the way that I have—narrative form, unencumbered, as much as possible, with references to the wider literature in the text itself, and using a language and form that Das, as the object of our gaze, could also recognize—arose out of discussions with fellow anthropologists in my own department, at Brunel University in London.[39] One of my colleagues, Andrew Beatty, was just completing his own narrative ethnography, *A Shadow Falls: In the Heart of Java*;[40] his answer to some of the epistemological conundrums I outlined above. Adopting a style more akin to that of a novel than a conventional monograph was not just a way of getting more people to read his book, even though he took seriously the importance of opening up anthropological findings and insights to wider audiences. Unlike the thematic structuring of more traditional ethnographies, a narrative approach also allowed him to "leave opaque what resists social analysis; it acknowledges the irreducible; it does not force an answer."[41] Telling it in story form enabled readers to grasp how Islamic fundamentalism might emerge in a place where tolerance of religious variation had once been the norm far better than an approach compelled to engage with pre-existing theoretical models.

Isak Niehaus, also a colleague, was at the same time writing an account of his own former research assistant, a South African teacher whose recent death, in 2005, he was still trying to make sense of. Like Das, Niehaus's interlocutor, Jimmy, a man he had worked with for 15 years, was also a close friend and colleague. And in his case, too, Jimmy's personal story helped to inform and enrich Niehaus's knowledge of wider themes pertinent to South Africa, from masculinities to witchcraft and misfortune, while responding to more personal curiosities. As was the case for Beatty, he had written extensively about these themes before:[42] in both cases, the change of genre allowed new things to be said in new ways, for theory to follow the narrative rather than—as is often the case—the other way around.

Writing Das's story had, by this time, been on my "to-do list" for several years, and my conversations with both Beatty and Niehaus about our respective projects convinced me that the story was one worth telling as well as helping me to think about the format it might take.

In respect of the latter, there were a number of forms in which my material could have been presented. Texts like *Viramma*, for example, appear entirely in the narrator's own words; edited, to be sure, but without direct reference to the anthropologists who facilitated the encounter or notes on how the data was gathered. Others, such as Alter, Crapanzano and Brown— all of whom I have referred to above—include large chunks, sometimes whole chapters, of their subjects' own words, but make clear their own role in the creation of the texts, acknowledging the power relations that not only made their encounters possible in the first place, but which shape the content and the form of the data. Brown, in common with anthropologists such as

Kirin Narayan,[43] also goes beyond what might be dubbed creative non-fiction to present elements of Mama Lola's history in the form of fictionalized short stories, a strategy which, she says, "allows me to tap a reservoir of casual and imagistic knowledge, which all people who have done fieldwork have but do not ordinarily use."[44] As Crapanzano demonstrates in *Tuhami*, the line between fact and fiction can anyway be a difficult one to draw: there were stories Tuhami told him which, while not literally true, revealed truths about him and the social worlds he lived in that cold reportage of facts alone could not.

In the following, I too use Das's own words as much as possible, but do not shy away from including my own interpretations (clearly identified as such) of what was going on, or, indeed, those offered by others I spoke to. Given that the story was created through our exchanges, it felt appropriate to maintain a sense this was a conversation rather than a monologue. I tried to avoid placing Das in unwitting dialogue with other ethnographic texts, although I have included references—where it felt appropriate—to a wider reading on significant topics that his story throws light upon. I did not, although I occasionally considered it, deliberately use fiction, although I did use language creatively to evoke scenes and situations that go beyond the content of the words we exchanged.[45] I also took the decision to change names, both of people and, sometimes, places and other minor identifying details. Das was initially ambivalent about this. "What does it matter?" he said when I discussed it with him. "My family can't read it, and they know all these things anyway!" But since some of the stories he told involved people whose consent could not be sought—cuckolded husbands, for instance, or the local politicians and officials he described as corrupt—it would have been unethical to identify them, however unlikely they might be to read the book. In the end Das came around to the idea, helping me to choose the names we gave to his family members and the other supporting roles in the cast of his life. He also read an entire draft of the manuscript—most of it on a twenty-four-hour train journey we took together to Mumbai, me passing on chapters as I proofread them—before I sent the text to the publisher for review. He queried a few minor factual details, which I corrected, but was satisfied with the overall thrust, even with the depictions of our disagreements. "That's how it happened," he shrugged. "People can make up their own minds whether I am good or bad, if the things I did were right or wrong. I don't mind what they think. At least *everything* is there, they have the full story."

There is, of course, no single "full story." There are, I am sure, many omissions in the following account, and Das, I have no doubt, is canny enough to exclude, or at to least temper, stories that he felt might show him in an entirely negative light or which might unnecessarily threaten our friendship. I imagine my own self-representations suffer the same failings.

Nor do my attempts to represent Das fairly fully mitigate the mostly unspoken differences in power between us. I, as a white westerner employed in a British University, had the resources to come in and out of Das's life, sometimes providing money and work, and serving, through the charity of which I was a trustee, as a conduit for funds that supported social welfare programs on which he and his family relied. Das did not have the same resources available to him. That we came to know each other at all, in the way that we did, is something inextricably rooted in larger colonial and missionary histories—what Alter calls a "hybrid history of encounter."[46] But, for all those caveats, it is, I think, a version of history worth telling. What follows is my attempt at making sense of it all and, in the process, of making sense of Das.

NOTES

1. To protect identities, names of people and some of the places mentioned in this book have been changed, although I have attempted to retain, as much as possible, the spirit of the originals.
2. R. C. Dogra, and U. Dogra, *Thought Provoking Hindu Names* (New Delhi: Star Publications, 2008).
3. See, for a more detailed discussion of my approach, James Staples, "Nuancing 'leprosy stigma' through ethnographic biography in South India," *Leprosy Review* 82, 2 (2011): 109–123. This is an approach which draws, in turn, on such works as George C. Rosenwald and Richard L. Ochberg, *Storied Lives: The Cultural Politics of Self-understanding* (New Haven: Yale University Press, 1992); Gelya Frank, "Anthropology and individual lives: the story of the life history and the life history of the story," *American Anthropologist*, 97 (1995):145–48; L.L. Langness and Gelya Frank, *Lives: An Anthropological Approach to Biography* (Novato, California: Chandler and Sharp Publishers, Inc. 1981); Charlotte, Linde, *Life Stories: The Creation of Coherence* (New York: Oxford University Press, 1993); and James L. Peacock and Dorothy C. Holland, "The Narrated Self: Life Stories in Process," *Ethos* 21, 4 (1993): 367–383.
4. Vikas Swarup, *Q & A* (London: Black Swan, 2006).
5. See, for discussion of the socio-historical background to leprosy, Rod Edmond, *Leprosy and Empire: a Medical and Cultural History* (Cambridge: Cambridge University Press, 2006); and—specifically in relation to leprosy in South India—Jane Buckingham, *Leprosy in Colonial South India* (London: Palgrave, 2002); de Bruin, H. M. *Leprosy in South India: Stigma and Strategies of Coping* (Pondy Paper in Social Sciences: Institute Francais de Pondicherry, 1996).
6. For an extended discussion of this see James Staples, *Peculiar People, Amazing Lives: Leprosy, Social Exclusion and Community Making in South India* (New Delhi: Orient Longman, 2007), 16–21, *et passim*. See also Jonathan Parry, "The marital history of 'A Thumb-Impression man,'" in *Telling Lives in India: Biography, Autobiography and Life History*, eds. David Arnold and Stuart Blackburn (Bloomington: Indiana University Press, 2004), 286.
7. I discuss the wider strategy of blaming the victim in James Staples, "Culture and Carelessness: constituting disability in South India," *Medical Anthropology Quarterly* 26, 4 (2012): 557–74. See also Leti Volpp, "Blaming culture for bad behaviour," *Yale Journal of Law and the Humanities* 12 (2000): 89–117, and Melissa Leach and James Fairhead, *Vaccine Anxieties: Global Science, Child Health and Society* (London: Earthscan, 2007). On "structural violence" see Paul Farmer, *Pathologies of Power: Health, Human Rights, and the New War on the Poor* (Berkeley: University of California Press, 2005).
8. A point well-made by David Arnold and Stuart Blackburn, "Introduction: Life Histories in India," in *Telling Lives in India: Biography, Autobiography and Life History*, eds. David Arnold and Stuart Blackburn (Bloomington: Indiana University Press, 2004), 5–6. See also Pat Caplan, "The transcendent subject? Biography as a medium for writing 'life and times,'" in

Extraordinary Encounters: Authenticity and the Interview, eds. Katherine Smith, James Staples and Nigel Rapport (Oxford: Berghahn, in press).

9. On the embodiment of caste, see Staples, *Peculiar People, Amazing Lives*, 133–134, 143–147; Susan Bayly, *Caste, Society and Politics in India from the Eighteenth Century to the Modern Age* (Cambridge: Cambridge University Press, 1999), 7; Hugo Gorringe and Irene Rafanell, "The Embodiment of Caste: Oppression, Protest and Change," *Sociology* 41, 1(2007): 97–114; or—on the embodiment of identities and status more generally in India—see Meredith Lindsay McGuire, " 'How to sit, how to stand': bodily praxis and the new urban middle class," in *A Companion to the Anthropology of India*, ed. Isabelle Clark-Decès (Wiley-Blackwell: Oxford, 2011), 117–136. For more on caste in contemporary India more generally—including critiques of the classic Dumontian position (Louis Dumont, *Homo Hierarchicus, the Caste System and its Implications* [Chicago and London: University of Chicago Press, 1980])—see C. J. Fuller, ed. *Caste Today* (Delhi: Oxford University Press, 1997); Dipankar Gupta, *Interrogating Caste* (New Delhi: Penguin Books India, 2000); Dipankar Gupta, ed. *Caste in Question: Identity or Hierarchy?* (New Delhi: Sage, 2004); Mary Searle-Chattterjee and Ursula Sharma, eds., *Contextualising Caste* (Oxford: Blackwell, 2004); and M. N. Srinivas, ed. *Caste: its Twentieth Century Avatar* (New Delhi: Penguin Books India, 1997). On more specific recent transformations (pertinent to the caste to which Das claims membership) see C. J. Fuller, "The modern transformation of an old elite: the case of the Tamil Brahmins," in *A Companion to the Anthropology of India*, ed. Isabelle Clark-Decès (Chichester: Wiley-Blackwell, 2011), 80–97.

10. On "embodied dispositions" I am influenced in particular by Pierre Bourdieu, *Outline of a Theory on Practice* (Cambridge: Cambridge University Press, 1972). For a straightforward account of Bourdieu's *habitus*—the embodiment of history—see Richard Jenkins, *Pierre Bourdieu* (London: Routledge, 1992), 66–102.

11. David Arnold and Stuart Blackburn, "Introduction: Life Histories in India," in *Telling Lives in India: Biography, Autobiography and Life History*, eds. David Arnold and Stuart Blackburn (Bloomington: Indiana University Press, 2004) 5–6.

12. Gelya Frank, *Venus on Wheels: Two Decades of Dialogue on Disability, Biography and Being Female in America* (Berkeley: California University Press, 2000).

13. See Roger Sanjek, "Anthropology's hidden colonialism: assistants and their ethnographers," *Anthropology Today* 9, 2 (April 1993): 13–18; and Luke Eric Lassiter, *The Chicago Guide to Collaborative Ethnography* (Chicago: Chicago University Press, 2005).

14. For additional reflection, see Staples, "Nuancing 'leprosy stigma' through ethnographic biography in South India," *Leprosy Review* 109–23; or James Staples, "An 'up and down life': understanding leprosy through biography," in *Extraordinary Encounters*, eds. Katherine Smith, James Staples and Nigel Rapport (Oxford: Berghahn, in press).

15. Tim Ingold, *The Perception of the Environment: Essays in Livelihood, Dwelling and Skill* (London: Routledge, 2000), Chapter 10.

16. Certeau, Michel de, "Walking in the City," chapter seven in *The Practice of Everyday Life* (California: University of California Press, 1984).

17. Tim Ingold and Jo Lee Vergunst (eds), *Ways of Walking: Ethnography and Practice on Foot* (Burlington, VT: Ashgate, 2008), 1.

18. Jeannette Marie Mageo, "Figurative Dream Analysis and U.S. Traveling Identities," *Ethnos* 34, 4 (2006): 480.

19. Seminal texts marking the "crisis of representation" in anthropology in the 1980s—and which anticipated the debates about styles of representation in the years ahead—include James Clifford and George Marcus (eds.) *Writing Culture: The Poetics and Politics of Ethnography* (Berkeley: University of California Press, 1985); George E. Marcus and Michael M. J. Fischer (eds.) *Anthropology as Cultural Critique: An Experimental Moment in the Human Sciences* (Chicago: University of Chicago Press, 1986); and James Clifford, "On Ethnographic Authority," *Representations* 1, 2 (1983):118–146.

20. Andrew Beatty, "How Did It Feel For You? Emotion, Narrative, and the Limits of Ethnography." *American Anthropologist*, 112, 3 (2010): 437.

21. Joseph Alter, *Knowing Dil Das: Stories of a Himalayan Hunter* (Philadelphia, University of Pennsylvania Press, 2000) xii.

22. John Chernoff, *Hustling is Not Stealing: Stories of an African Bar Girl* (Chicago: University of Chicago Press, 2003).

23. Bronislaw Malinowski, *Argonauts of the Western Pacific: An Account of Native Enterprise and Adventure in the Archipelagoes of Melanesian New Guinea* (London: Routledge and Kegan Paul, 1922).

24. Paul Radin, *Crashing Thunder: The Autobiography of an American Indian* (Michigan: Michigan University Press, 1999 [1926]).

25. Leo W. Simmons (ed.) *Sun Chief: The Autobiography of a Hopi Indian* (New Haven: Yale University Press, 1942).

26. See, for critiques of the Native American narrated autobiography genre, Michelle Burnham, "'I Lied All the Time': Trickster Discourse and Ethnographic Authority in 'Crashing Thunder,'" *American Indian Quarterly*, 22, 4 (1988) 469–484 (which focuses specifically on Radin's pioneering volume) and Arnold Krupat, *For Those Who Came After: A Study of Native American Autobiography* (Berkeley: University of California Press, 1985).

27. Mary Smith, *Baba of Karo: A Woman of the Muslim Hausa* (New Haven: Yale University Press. 1981 [1954]).

28. Sidney W. Mintz, *Worker in the Cane: A Puerto Rican Life History* (New Haven: Yale University Press, 1960).

29. Vincent Crapanzano, *Tuhami: Portrait of a Moroccan* (Chicago: University of Chicago Press, 1980).

30. See Bruce T. Grindal and Frank A. Salamone (eds.) *Bridges to Humanity: Narratives on Fieldwork and Friendship* (Long Grove, Illinois: Waveland Press, 2006).

31. Karen McCarthy Brown, *Mama Lola: A Vodou Priestess in Brooklyn* (Berkeley: University of California Press, 1991).

32. Ibid: 9.

33. Ibid: 12.

34. James M. Freeman, *Untouchable: an Indian Life History* (London: Allen and Unwin, 1979).

35. Alter, *Knowing Dil Das.*

36. Vasant Moon, *Growing Up Untouchable in India: a Dalit Autobiography* (Landham, Maryland: Rowman and Littlefield, 2001).

37. Viramma, Josiane Racine and Jean-Luc Racine. *Viramma: Life of an Untouchable,* Translated by Will Hobson (London: Verso, 1997).

38. Although, unlike its French version, the English translation of *Viramma* includes no detail on how the material for the book was gathered, a subsequent book chapter provides this detail: see Josiane Racine, and Jean-Luc Racine, "Beyond Silence: A Dalit Life History in South India. In *Telling Lives in India: Biography, Autobiography and Life History,* edited by David Arnold and Stuart Blackburn (Bloomington: Indiana University Press, 2004) 252–280.

39. Older influences, now I think about it, were the texts that got me interested in anthropology in the first place: Nigel Barley's *The Innocent Anthropologist: Notes from a Mud Hut* (Prospect Heights, Illinois: Waveland Press, 2000 [1983]) was—back in 1984—the first book I read by an anthropologist; Claude Lévi-Strauss's older and more substantial *Tristes Tropiques* (English translation by John and Doreen Weightman, New York: Atheneum, 1973 [1955]) likewise evoked for me the process of fieldwork—and showed why it was important to our understanding—in a way that other classics, for all their theoretical elegance, did not. E. E. Evans-Pritchard's *The Nuer: a Description of the Models of Livelihood and Political Institutions of a Nilotic People* (Oxford: Oxford University Press, 1940), is a good example of the latter.

40. Andrew Beatty, *A Shadow Falls: In the Heart of Java* (London: Faber and Faber, 2009).

41. Andrew Beatty, "How Did It Feel For You? Emotion, Narrative, and the Limits of Ethnography." *American Anthropologist*, 112, 3 (2010): 438.

42. See Isak Niehaus, *Witchcraft, power and politics: exploring the occult in the South African Lowveld* (London: Pluto Press, 2001); Andrew Beatty, *Varieties of Javanese religion: an anthropological account* (Cambridge: Cambridge University Press, 1999); and *Society and exchange in Nias* (Oxford: Oxford University Press, 1992).

43. Kirin Narayan, *Love, Stars and All That* (New York: Pocket Books, 1994). See also her memoir, *My Family and Other Saints* (Chicago: University of Chicago Press, 2007) as an exemplar of creative non-fiction that draws on anthropological insights.

44. Brown, *Mama Lola*, 18.

45. See John van Maanen's *Tales of the Field: On Writing Ethnography* (University of Chicago Press, 1988), for useful discussion on how anthropologists use style to convey meaning in their texts. I also drew inspiration from Kirin Narayan's *Alive in the Writing: Crafting Ethnography in the Company of Chekhov* (Chicago: Chicago University Press, 2012).

46. Alter, *Knowing Dil Das,* 165.

Chapter One

Beginnings

Das was not quite one of "midnight's children," the fictional title Salman Rushdie gave in his book of the same name to those born literally on the cusp of Indian independence at midnight on August 14, 1947.[1] He was, though, part of that first post-colonial generation. One and a half thousand miles from the fanfares of Delhi, where, just three months earlier, India had cut its last official ties with Britain and became an independent republic on January 26, Das entered the world on May 3, 1950, born in a small village in Thanjavur District, central Tamil Nadu, in the Kaveri river delta.

We visited his village together in August 2009, more than half a century after he left it, as part of the process of gathering together material from which to tell Das's life story. It also gave us several days of interview time uninterrupted by his immediate family and current neighbours. Long train journeys and bus rides were the best opportunities I had to put Das's narrative under scrutiny.

In response to the village, Das was struck by how familiar it still seemed. "Bit by bit, the place where I lived came back to me, even though I was only six or seven years old when we left," he told me when we returned to our lodgings the evening after our visit. We were discussing what he had made of the place. "In those days," he said, slightly wistfully, "it was full of people, and there were always lots of children. It seemed quieter now than it had done."

Other things had remained the same. The pond where he and his peers had bathed, and on the edges of which their mothers washed clothes, was still there and in regular use, even if there were no children playing marbles on its banks any longer. And the residential clusters, organized by caste, were still where Das remembered them as being, along with the temple and the school.

We stayed in a cheap hotel near the bus stand in Kumbakonam, the major temple pilgrimage town where Das also lived for several years after his family migrated from the village. It was two local bus rides—an hour and a half or so away—from the roadside track that had eventually led us, on foot, into the place of his birth. Although we arrived there early in the morning, having set out straight after our hurried breakfast of masala dosas—crisp South Indian pancakes, stuffed with potato curry—it was already hot. The monsoon, if it ever came at all that year, had not yet reached Tamil Nadu. But the parched pathway before us was at least shaded by towering coconut palms, and after following it half a mile or so in from the road, Das's old elementary school finally came into view. A few small children had already gathered together in the courtyard, gazing up at us inquisitively as we passed by, even though classes would not begin for another couple of hours. It was here that Das had studied for two years, sitting with the other Brahmins on the front benches. "It was all mixed," he recalled, looking up at the shrine, guarded on either side by two stone-carved oxen, which dominated the compound. "No-one had to sit outside or anything, which is what I think happened in some villages, where they wouldn't let the lowest castes come in, but the seating in the class rooms was ordered by caste. The teachers were mostly Brahmins, and they'd allocate the front benches to the higher castes." Any further concessions, his words implied, would have been taking egalitarianism too far.

A few hundred yards further along the track, we reached the Brahmin enclave where Das had lived, set away from the streets occupied by the Vaisyas—the trading castes—and, beyond them, the rest. True to his earlier descriptions of it, at the top of the wide, tree-lined street was a temple, and there were about fifteen households on either side. The Iyers (Shaivas, or followers of the God Shiva)—which included Das's family—lived on one side of the street, and the Iyengars (originally members of the break-away Vaishnavite sect), on the other.

In the 1950s, most of the houses, and certainly the one Das lived in, had been constructed from mud, but now all of them had been transformed into brick built *pakka* dwellings, topped with the distinctive red curved tiles common to the area. The houses were also laid out in what, he told me, was a typical Tamil Brahmin style. Each had a verandah shaded by the overhang of the roof with a raised platform or two, designed for sleeping on, at the front. Beyond the rooms leading directly off the verandah would be a relatively large, privately enclosed courtyard, one half sheltered by a roof, the other open to the elements. The covered side, in all the houses we entered, accommodated the *puja* area at one end—a cluster of garland bedecked idols and burning incense arranged on a small niche, vital for everyday religious rituals—and beds and chairs at the other. The two spaces were separated with a large, flat wooden swing, suspended from the rafters on thick ropes, in the centre. I had seen similar seats in the city bungalows of some of Das's wealthier relatives in Chennai: "Brahmins like them," he told me, as if by way of explanation. Behind the courtyards were storerooms, large enough to retain a family's personal crop of rice, de-husked and sacked-up, and then hot, dark kitchens, the walls blackened from cooking over open fires. Toilets and wells were situated in the backyards beyond.

Das's own house had been much simpler: two rooms with mud walls but a similarly tiled roof, and a small verandah at the front on which the family usually slept. There was a brick built house on the plot now, newly renovated, but Das remembered the place well. We were standing there with the *Munsif* (village headman), who had volunteered to show us around, when the location also nudged his own memory. "Yes!" he said suddenly, looking at Das. "You had a sister, but she had something . . . something wrong with her legs, was it? They stood her here, on this spot, in a bucket, I think, filled with sand . . ."

'Yes, yes!' came Das's reply, his head nodding up and down in excitement at their sudden mutual recognition, however blurred, of one another's families. The two men were roughly the same age. "That was her. She had some kind of weakness, maybe it was from polio, I'm not sure, but yes, this is where we stood her in that thing, it was to help strengthen her legs, to teach her how to walk." Talking faster now, the two men reeled off names of other villagers and people to whom they were distantly related in an attempt to place one another more firmly. The connections were vague, for which Das was, I think, grateful—he did not have to explain about his leprosy—but they had been made, and the *Munsif* visibly relaxed after that moment of recognition had taken place. We were no longer strangers.

The *Munsif* took us back to his house. There, the morning *Sandhya Vandhanam* rituals, during which the male householders had anointed their foreheads with their distinctive horizontal stripes of ash, were already completed, but the men had not yet left for work. These days, the *Munsif* told us, they ran a factory and a coconut plantation on their land toward the main road. We were seated on plastic armchairs in the shade of the inner courtyard with two of his younger brothers to keep us company, and he sent the wife of one of them to prepare us fresh coffee, milky, sweet and aromatic, which arrived some time later in small, shiny stainless steel cups, held within deep stainless steel saucers. "It's the way we Brahmins drink coffee in Tamil Nadu," Das told me proudly, back at the hotel that evening, as we shared a bottle of beer in very un-Brahmin-like fashion, distributed between two flimsy plastic cups. He had explained to me the particularities of Brahmin coffee drinking several times over the years, usually when we were eating at a Brahmin run restaurant he liked in Chennai, but he was enjoying the opportunity this visit had presented to relish his Brahmin-ness, so I let him tell me again. "They always serve it in two vessels, the cup and the bowl, so that you can mix the coffee together with the sugar and get it to just the right temperature before you drink it," he said. "The temperature is important, so you can just pour it in without the cup touching your lips, and that keeps the cup clean."

"So would I have ruined that cup for them?" I asked, worried now that I would have been seen as violating their purity. My lips had met the cup with every sip, and—beyond savouring the smell and taste of freshly ground South Indian coffee, a substance increasingly replaced with instant brews on street stalls—I had not given it much thought. My fieldwork to date had mostly been with low-caste, economically poor people, many of them converted Christians with leprosy who, understandably, had chosen to reject this kind of thinking altogether. In those situations, demonstrating a willingness to accept food and to use the same vessels as they did was much more important. Considerations of purity and pollution had mainly been confined to what I had read in ethnographies about Hindu India.[2] I knew about these things in theory but they had a kind of mythical quality about them. I was not used to coming across them in everyday life.

"No, not these days!" Das reassured me. "They'll just wash it. I already said to them, asked if they were sure before we went in, told them you were a foreigner, not a Brahmin, but they were 'no, no, he can take.'"

It reminded him: "I took Apitha [his Muslim next door neighbour], Fauzia's daughter, to my mother's house in Madras a few years ago, she was just eight or nine I think, and she'd never seen coffee served like that before. I said she needed to make it cool and I showed her how to drink it. When she came back to the village she was laughing about it in our street and demonstrating to everyone how she had to drink it!"

Das enjoyed these kinds of reminisces because they reinforced to him how he was different: they demonstrated that he knew things other people in the places he had lived subsequently did not know. It was not so much that he saw himself as superior to others. His friends came from a wide range of caste and religious backgrounds, and he could speak happily with most people we encountered in fieldwork contexts, from people begging on the streets to hospital consultants. It was one of the reasons I liked working with him. Self-consciousness of his caste status did, however, give him a confidence in himself and a positive identity that he was comfortable with; one that he also knew brought respect from others.

It was perhaps for this reason that earlier, more synoptic accounts of his life history made his start in life appear particularly auspicious. He was, after all, born a Tamil Brahmin, and several of his extended kin group—his male second cousins, especially—appeared to have done very well for themselves, moving on to prestigious jobs in Dubai, Germany, the U.S. and the UK. Had it not been for the onset of leprosy, such stories implied, Das might also have that kind of life. He had been set up with a job in Bombay after leaving school by one of his relatives, a senior tax inspector, and his own father, until he too got leprosy, had run a series of apparently successful meals hotels.

Such stories, however, obscured more than they revealed, positive elements over-egged as a device to highlight how damaging social reactions to leprosy can be. It was only because he contracted the disease and the associated shame that forced him to walk away from his former life, such stories implied; only leprosy that led him to virtual destitution at one point, rather than, say, to becoming a chartered accountant in west London like one of his cousins. But compelling though those narratives are—particularly to charities that want to show the world why leprosy remains such a social problem—Das's start in life was never quite as auspicious as that of his more prosperous relatives.

Firstly, Brahmin though he was, he was born into what was already the poorest branch of his family. His mother, Subbalakshmi, was an only child whose father had died before she was born. Her own mother, although she had an acre or two of land, was consequently poorer than she would have been had her husband lived and had she produced at least one son. She was almost certainly the least prosperous of all her sibling group. They got by: the land yielded just enough rice to sustain them, but there was no accumulation of wealth going on in the years she raised her daughter. Neither was there money for a dowry, and—as she had no sons to stay and care for her— Subbalakshmi's mother was anyway not keen on losing her daughter to another family.

In another branch of the family—the connections between them sufficiently distant as not to be picked up in my rudimentary family tree—Tejaswami, a schoolmaster, was looking for a match for his eldest son, Gajavakra. His other three sons were all reasonably well-placed: the second one was undertaking training to become a Tamil *Pandit*; one had followed in his father's footsteps and trained as a school teacher; and the third had his own small tea hotel. Gajavakra, however, had "always been a bit of a wanderer," as Das put it. He was bright but had not attended much school, and needed, his father thought, to get married in order to settle him down. But what respectable Brahmin family could be persuaded to take this boy without qualifications or a job?

Subbalakshmi offered the ideal solution. Her family could not offer a dowry—so could not be too choosy in selecting a husband—but her mother did have a little land to leave behind and no sons. Also, because Gajavakra could go and live in his wife's village with her he would be taken off his father's hands. This was unusual: for Hindus, the bride is considered a gift, taken on by her husband's family.[3] Connections with the bride's family are subsequently restricted, and the couple are expected to live in the groom's natal residence. Variations on this were far from unheard of, however, and I knew of several cases of husbands going to live with their wives' families when circumstances demanded it. Gajavakra's residential arrangements might not have been looked upon as ideal, but they were not exceptional either.

The couple married as planned when Subbalakshmi was nineteen, Gajavakra moving to the village from his natal town of Udayarpalayam in a neighbouring district. By the time Das was born a couple of years later in 1950, Gajavakra had begun working in a small meals hotel in Anaikarai, a small island in the Kaveri river basin connected to the main land via bridges, about four miles away from the village. He walked there early every morning, returning only at about ten o'clock each evening, so Das's earliest memories of his father were more of his absence than his presence.

It is difficult to get much of an impression from Das of what his mother was like, either. Perhaps, because of all the years they were apart later on, and their sporadic contact in the years up until her death in 2007, his own memories of her were also blurred. Or perhaps it was because he saw her, quite simply, as his mother, a relatively straightforward categorization on which he saw little need for deeper reflection. Certainly, on the two occasions that I met her, by which time she was living with a wealthier female relative in Chennai, Parvathi, who she cared for, Das's mother mostly hovered in the background, a physically slight figure who stayed out of all but the most perfunctory of conversations. She greeted us, gracefully and softly, asked after her son's wife and children's health, and then withdrew to the back of the room until it was time for her to prepare and serve food. In this she proved herself an attentive host, quietly cajoling everyone to eat more. The much larger figure of her companion, meanwhile, held forth from her perch on the swing in the centre of the room.

Asked about his memories of his mother, Das said, simply: "My mother was not educated. She was very innocent, not easy to anger, and although sometimes she would lose her temper with us children if we misbehaved, she'd just beat me lightly on the head, but not even that very much."

"There were no other special things about my mother," he went on, struggling to find things to say. "Cooking, staying in the house . . . that's what she did. Later, when she moved to stay with this other family, with Parvathi, she learned things: English words, about going out and purchasing groceries in the bazaar. When she was with us, even when we moved to the cities, she wouldn't go out and purchase things. We, the men, bought all the groceries and other things. But when she was with that other family she learned all those things."

She also, Das made clear, knew how to behave as a Brahmin in ways that his own wife, who was not of his caste, never could. When I asked if there were any similarities between the two women, he shook his head and tutted. It was a self-evidently dim-witted question. "My mother, she was born into a Brahmin family, and even though they were poor, she knew the culture and how to behave in a certain way. Even though she was not educated she knew how to move, how to talk to her husband and her children. She learned these things as she grew up, very gradually, so they are natural to her. Someone who hasn't come from that background can't learn those things later on. It's not their fault, but they can't, it's not in them." Caste, in Das's worldview, was very much embodied.

Unlike his wife, who was partial to mutton, Das's mother also knew how to cook like a Brahmin, even when money for food was scarce. Their land, when they still had it, would provide a couple of sacks of rice a year, and around the sides of the house they grew aubergines and tomatoes, and a few green leafy vegetables. They also consumed parts of their banana trees other than the fruit: "the stem, it looks a bit like a tube light, we'd cut that up and make a curry or a fried side dish—very good for the digestion—and the flower, too, you can cook with lentils and coconut. Even the leaves got used as plates for outside people to eat from." This also meant, of course, that outsiders could not pollute their own plates.[4]

Like the meals she served me in Madras (by then renamed Chennai) many years later, they would centre around rice, served first with *sambar*—a soup-like aromatic lentil and vegetable stew—and one or two vegetable dishes, or a *papad*, usually fried in ghee; then *rasam*—a peppery broth made from tamarind water or tomatoes; and then, with the last of the rice, curd or buttermilk and pickles, preserved from limes and mangoes grown on their own land. The meal would become more complex, with additional courses interspersed, on special occasions or in more affluent households, and the sambar would become thinner and the vegetable side dishes fewer in leaner times, but the basic structure of the meal always, at least in Das's memories, remained the same. Most of the families where he lived now ate more simply: a single curry and rice, then curd or pickle, reduced, in some households, to little more than rice flavoured with hot pickles or chilli powder when money was particularly scarce. Celebratory meals there were distinguishable not by the complexity of their courses but by the addition of meat, cooked in spicy *masalas*, and the rice transformed into an oily *pulao* or infused with coconut rather than simply boiled.

Other commensal rules were also followed more rigidly in his mother's house than in his current home, and although Das conceded that these rules—such as the women eating separately and later than the men—were not caste specific, adherence to them was much stronger in Brahmin households. "If my mother had her menses, for example, she wouldn't even come into the house," he said. "Women, in that condition, would always stay in a separate part, eat from a separate plate, drink from a separate cup. In my village, normally they'd have a small room on the verandah, and she'd sit there. If she wanted water, we'd pour it for her; if she wanted food we'd bring the

food and put it there for her. If the serving spoon touched her plate we'd need
to take it away and wash it."

"These customs are not followed so much in the other castes," he went
on, warming to this theme. "When the husband dies, his widow will shave
her head and needs to wear white clothes, maybe only *khadi* [hand spun
cotton] cloth, if she's very observant. Old ladies wear *khadi* anyway, in the
Brahmin castes. Nowadays, of course, they won't bother so much, even very
devoted women like Parvathi, who my mother lived with. She stopped wearing a kumkum and flowers in her hair after her husband died, but she didn't
wear only white. My mother didn't wear white either, but she also stopped
flowers and removed her bangles and all that."[5]

As Brahmins, they also maintained hereditary service relationships with
other caste groups, although, for Das's family at least, these were already
dwindling by the 1950s.[6] "We had our own barber who came to cut our hair,"
he said, "and we'd give him paddy, no money, I don't think. And there was
also a priest who would come for the family when we called him, but although he also took rice and other gifts, by that time they'd also started
charging money for their services." They also had someone to take care of
the land, a fairly distant relative who also lived in the village, and Das's
mother helped them—"to clean the house and other things"—in exchange.

In terms of Hindu religious rituals, Das's memories are fuzzier. He had,
after all, spent the last twenty-five years in a predominantly Christian village,
and over the decade or so prior to that had followed a more or less secular
lifestyle, so religion was less embodied in Das's everyday actions than it was
for, say, the *Munsif* and his family. Even when they lived in the village,
however, they were not the most devout of families. "It was like this," he
explained. "Nowadays, I'm a converted Christian, but I'm not going much to
church, although some Christians there attend church three or more times a
week. I was the same kind of Hindu as I am a Christian: believing, but not
going that deeply."

"In every family, of course, there must be affection shown toward God,
with at least one or two older people, usually the women, doing the *pujas* for
all the family. Not everyone needs to be involved in the same way. My father
wasn't there much in the house in the morning, he went early to the hotels to
work and came late at night, so I never remember seeing him doing any
pujas. But my uncle, say, he would do. In our house, we'd follow Subram-
maniam, the son of Shiva. Our family was devoted, just not very deeply. But
we went to temple and other things: my mother would go every Friday, at
least, and we'd attend at festival and special *puja* times, but there are some
people who will go everyday."

Das's own recollections of attending the temple were during festivals:
"During the cold season, in the month of Maargazhi [mid-December to mid-
January], they'd do *Bhajanas* (devotional songs) at the temple. I remember

because *pongal* [a sweet festival dish of rice, cooked with lentils, dried fruit and cashew nuts] would be prepared there and served to everyone, and I'd go in order to eat it! Everyone went, or at least the men, although I don't remember my father going . . . maybe he'd already left by then?"

It was not entirely clear when Gajavakra first left the family, or whether his departure to Kumbakonam much preceded that of Das, his mother and their children, although Das recalls that he was around when his sister— Kaveri—was born in 1954. She was, as the *Munsif* had recalled, "affected." In Das's words, she had "very thin legs and a protruding belly, and she couldn't walk properly." They had massaged cod liver oil into her legs, and she spent a lot of time propped up in sand in a drum, which enabled her to stand and so strengthened her legs. She "slowly learned to walk" through repeating this daily ritual, although never, Das thinks, in the usual way.

The precise timing of his father's departure from the village is uncertain, but it must have been sometime between 1954 and 1956, because it was in 1956 that his mother received word that her husband was sick with cholera in the Government hospital in Kumbakonam. That, although not even Gajavakra knew it by then, was not all that was wrong with him. The entire household—Das, his maternal grandmother, mother and sister—packed up their things, left the land in the care of the relative who had anyway been looking after of it, and shifted to the town to look after him, and to be with him, or so they thought, on his release from hospital. They were not aware of it at the time, but they would never return to live in the village again.

NOTES

1. Salman Rushdie, *Midnight's Children* (Penguin Books, 1991).
2. For the classic argument that Hindu society is structured around distinctions between relative levels of purity and impurity see, for example, Louis Dumont, and David Pocock, "Pure and Impure," *Contributions to Indian Sociology*, 3 (1959): 9–39; Dumont, *Homo Hierarchicus*; Frederique Apfell Marglin, "Power, Purity and Pollution: Aspects of the Caste System Reconsidered," *Contributions to Indian Sociology* (NS) 11, 2 (1977): 245–270; McKim Marriott and Ronald Inden, "Toward an Ethnosociology of South Asian Caste Systems," in *The New Wind: Changing Identities in South Asia*, ed. K. David (The Hague: Mouton, 1977), 227–238; Michael Moffatt, *An Untouchable Community in South India: Structure and Consensus* (Princeton, N.J.: Princeton University Press, 1979); Susan S. Bean, "Toward a Semiotics of 'Purity' and 'Pollution' in India," *American Ethnologist*, 8, 3 (1981): 575– 595.
3. See, for example, Lina M. Fruzzetti, *The Gift of a Virgin: Women, Marriage, and Ritual in a Bengali Society* (Delhi: Oxford University Press, 1990).
4. For classic discussions on pollution and purity in relation to Indian commensality, see McKim Marriott, "Caste ranking and food transactions: A matrix analysis," in *Structure and Change in Indian Society*, eds M. Singer, and B. S. Cohn (Chicago: Aldine, 1968), 133–71; Adrian Mayer, *Caste and Kinship in Central India: A Village and Its Region* (London: Routledge, 1960); Andre Béteille, *Caste, Class and Power: Changing Patterns of Social Stratification in a Tanjore Village* (Oxford: Oxford University Press, 1996); Robert Deliége, *The Untouchables of India*, trans. Nora Scott (Oxford: Berg, 1999). For a more recent overview— which sets out to nuance the linear hierarchy implied by commensal rules—see James Staples,

"'Go on, just try some!': Meat and Meaning-Making among South Indian Christians," *South Asia: Journal of South Asian Studies* (NS) 31, 1 (2008): 36–55.

5. For comparison, see Sarah Lamb, *White Saris and Sweet Mangoes: Aging, Gender, and Body in North India* (Berkeley: University of California Press, 2000).

6. For more on *jajmani*—the system of hereditary service relationships that Das was referring to—see Peter Mayer, "Inventing village tradition: the late nineteenth century origins of the north Indian 'jajmani system,'" *Modern Asian Studies* 27 (1993) 357–395; C. J. Fuller, "Misconceiving the grain heap: a critique of the concept of the 'Indian jajmani system,'" in *Money and the Morality of Exchange*, eds. Jonathan Parry and Maurice Bloch (Cambridge: Cambridge University Press, 1989), 33–63.

Chapter Two

To the City

It may have been because we arrived so early in the morning—about 5am—but getting down from the bus and stretching our legs it felt pleasantly cooler, and the air clearer, than it had done the evening before when we had set off from Chennai. Compared to the town where Das now lived, or even to Vijayawada, the closest nearby town in terms of size to Kumbakonam, there was also a palpable sense of calm and order. We were greeted with newly swept roads and an orderly grid of market stalls displaying immaculate pyramids of fruit—oranges, apples and sweet limes, carefully arranged between layers of magenta pink tissue paper—alongside South Indian sweetmeats topped with slithers of edible silver, almonds or pistachios, neatly displayed within shiny glass cabinets. It was like an image from a glossy tourist guide. Between the stalls were also the giveaway signs that this was a temple town: carts selling garlands of heavily scented jasmine and marigolds, coconuts, incense sticks and the other paraphernalia of Hindu worship.[1] The sweets and the fruit, too, were probably sold mostly as *prasadam*: food symbolically offered to the temple deities before being fed to devotees.

As one might also expect of a major temple town, the roads stretching out from the bus stand were replete with lodges, hotels and cheap eating places to accommodate the pilgrims, so we had no difficulty in finding a simple room to stay in over night. Nor did we face the suspicious inquisitiveness sometimes invoked by a white foreigner and an Indian national trying to book hotel rooms together. The receptionist simply looked up, smiled pleasantly and, without asking, wrote "temple tourism" in the "reason for stay" column in his hotel register.

We were not far—about fifteen-minutes on foot, as it transpired when we walked there later that afternoon—from Pachaiyappa Mudali Street, the location where Das, his grandmother, mother and sister had rented accommodation when they arrived here in 1956. One of Das's grandmother's cousins—her father's brother's son—already lived in Kumbakonam, so he had been able to find them a place to stay ahead of their arrival from the village in a suitable Brahmin street. These days the house, number seven, is painted Krishna blue, a two-storey red-tiled brick building sandwiched between two taller houses. There was a red motorbike outside, but no other signs of life through the small windows, and a large padlock fastened the door. "It was more like a village house in those days," Das told me as we stood outside looking up at his old home. "The place was divided into six portions, each one rented out to a different family." Both he and his brother Chandra Prakash, who was born there in 1960, remember it as "Single Street," so called because houses were built only down one side of the road, the other taken up with a large rectangular water tank, now entirely dried out.

Gajavakra should have joined them there once he was released from hospital, but, as Das recalls it, he never did. Instead, he took off, as they discovered later, to the town of Kurur, one hundred miles east of Kumbakonam, where he ended up working in another tea hotel. Quite why he left at that point was unclear. It could have been simply a continuation of his tendency toward flight, although Das suspects Gajavakra already knew by then that he had leprosy, and was not ready to face his family with the news.

Whatever Gajavakra's reasons, the rest of his immediate family, having already set up home there and enrolled Das in school, stayed on in Kumbakonam. One of Das's earliest memories of the place was how, aged around three, his sister Kaveri had once followed behind him when he went out to the bazaar without being spotted by other family members. He had not noticed her either, and, unable to keep up, she soon lost her way in the narrow streets of the market, where she was discovered crying by one of the coffee bean merchants. He sat her down on his wooden counter and remedied her tears with sweet peanut clusters from a nearby tea stall. It was there, sitting contentedly and enjoying sugary snacks, that Das, who had returned home to discover her missing, eventually found her.

The next time Das talked to me about Kaveri was to recount the story of her contracting what he thought was probably small pox (*ammai*). "She was sick and stayed in the house for about ten days, and then my grandmother came down with it too. They seemed to be getting better, but after another couple of weeks, I came back home to find everyone crying and wailing. My sister had died." His grandmother also died a few days later, leaving Das and his mother alone.

If life was difficult then Das did not seem to be particularly aware of it. "My mother managed with the rice she'd brought from the land—it still produced a few sacks a year for us—and I think she did some work: grinding flour for breakfast stalls, cutting vegetables, things she could do from home. She cooks normally, no? So by doing a bit more she could make some extra income. We were poor, but running: the rice would come and mostly we'd have enough to eat."

Das also had support from the neighbors at number four, whom he got to know quite well over the next few years. An older woman called Visrantamma, who suffered from asthma and spent a lot of her time in bed, stayed there with her son, Shankar, who was studying for his Bachelor's degree. They were Vaishnavas, followers of the God Vishnu, and had left behind most of their family back in their village, although there were a couple of cousins also at Das's school. "He wasn't that clever," recalled Das of Shankar. "But they'd come to Kumbakonam from their village so he could study, and they were quite wealthy, I think."

When Shankar was at college his mother would sometimes call Das in from where he was playing cricket with other neighbours in the street to run errands for her: collecting vegetables and other groceries from the market or, sometimes, buying *idlis* (steamed spongy dumplings of fermented rice and pulses) and other breakfast items from nearby tiffin stalls. It meant he also got a share of the food and, sometimes, could keep the change, spending it on sweets and trips to the cinema. In addition, Visrantamma and her son took an interest in Das's education, buying him school textbooks, paper and pencils when he needed them. "I went to school fairly regularly," Das said. "I'd go there and sit in the class and listen in, but not much more than that. If there was an exam, I attended and wrote down what I could remember, but I never once prepared. I'd just take my bath at home as normal and go into school and write the papers. And I'd get 45 or 50 percent and pass, that's all. But apart from that family who helped me, nobody else had much of an interest. My father wasn't around, and my mother, well, she was uneducated herself, so couldn't have helped me much anyway, but she was also too busy with looking after the house and other things."

Das probably learned as much sitting in Visrantamma's house as he did at Kumbakonam High School. The three of them, he remembered, would spend evenings playing Monopoly and, sometimes, Carrom board, the radio tuned in to an English language station in the background. It was from listening to cricket matches on the radio, Das thinks, that he learned to speak English so fluently. "The nickname they gave me," he said, "was 'And-he's-out,' because that's what they used to hear me shouting every time I bowled a cricket ball to one of my friends in the street. It was something I'd heard on the radio. So if they saw me coming they'd call, 'Here comes And-he's-out!,' and beckon me to come inside and sit with them."

He never saw a game of cricket onscreen until the mid-1980s, "but it didn't matter. We'd listen all the time to the commentary, imagine in our heads what was going on, and then copy what they said when we were playing. You'd hear the commentator say, 'and the ball's cruising down the middle'—that was a line I repeated a lot—and we'd try to do it ourselves in the streets." In 1964 or 1965, he recalled, there was a five-day match in Coimbatore. Mansoor Ali Khan, the then captain of the Indian cricket team, was one of the stars, and Das had tuned in avidly every day. "We were visiting my mother's relatives there," he told me, "as we did with my mother in the holiday seasons. And when there were big matches on, everyone would listen."

Gajavakra crops up now and again in Das's narrative, his returns and departures providing useful temporal markers along the way. He wrote to them from Kurur, and the family also got word to him when his daughter and mother-in-law died. He returned, first, in 1959, and set up a small tiffin hotel selling idlis, dosas and tea, on a small plot towards the edge of town. Das and I walked there too, but the area was in the process of being redeveloped, and the buildings there now bore no resemblance to the single storey shack that Gajavakra had once traded from. He stayed long enough to be there for the arrival of his second son, Chandra Prakash, in 1960, but left shortly afterwards. The hotel was making a loss, and when he could no longer cover his debts, he absconded once more. A Malayali couple who had been working for him, presumably realizing that they no longer had jobs, sold off the cooking vessels and anything else he had left behind, before taking off themselves. This time Gajavakra travelled further, around 700 miles north, ending up in Jagdalpur, Bastar District, in what is now Chhattisgarh. "He had no history there, no relatives or debtors he would run into," Das said when I questioned why he chose that particular location. "Like me, he'd have got on a train and seen where it took him." Once there, probably after working for a while in other people's food businesses, he started another small idli business with a local friend he made there, Palani. He was away for a couple of years, returning in 1963 and then working in a variety of meals hotels to support the family.

Back in Single Street, life went on much as before. For Das, at least from his perspective nearly forty-five years later, it was a time of Carrom board, Monopoly, and cricket in the street with friends, most of whom he no longer even remembers the names of. "We weren't thinking about girls and that kind of thing back in those days," Das claimed. "Even at school, you didn't get the kind of ragging that you read about happening now, teasing boys about being in love with particular girls and the like, it was very rare, I think, even though it was a co-educational school." And so life went on for Das, his new brother and his mother, at least until 1965, when Gajavakra decided to shift the entire family to Madras.

Gajavakra went to Madras first, alone. He had had enough of working for other people and, despite the problems he had faced in making a profit from his own enterprises he was ready to try again. Parvathi, Das's mother's first cousin (her mother's brother's daughter), the woman she eventually lived with, was already staying in Madras with her husband and children at the time, and this was probably important in Gajavakra's choice of location. Parvathi had grown up in the same village as Subbalakshmi and, although their fortunes had diverged significantly, the two women always remained close. Like Subbalakshmi, Parvathi had married a relative, Subrahmanyam. Unlike Subbalakshmi's husband Gajavakra, however, Subrahmanyam had done well at school and became "well settled," acquiring a government job and working his way through the ranks eventually to become a chief tax commissioner. By the time Das was born, he had already been posted to Vizags, the naval town at the northernmost peak of Andhra Pradesh, and, during much of the time Das's family were in Kumbakonam, had been living closer-by in Coimbatore, where Das and his mother spent the summer holidays. Parvathi had helped her cousin financially in the past, and she helped again now, advancing Gajavakra some money to start his new small business and find somewhere to live.

Initially, he rented a room in what Das described as a "slum area": a thatched hut in a multi-caste street, where he apparently lived alongside people from scheduled castes and scheduled tribes—the official terms for those formerly known as untouchables, and, in Das's vocabulary, always abbreviated to the initials SC and ST or, more elliptically, "*those* people." His mother would not have objected to such a living arrangement, Das thought—and she passed no comment on it when they arrived—but his father thought it was unsuitable for them. Soon after the family joined him, in late 1965 or early 1966, he found alternative accommodation in Jothi Ramalingam Street: a single room in a terraced, single storey row with its own verandah at the front and shared toilet facilities.

It was from here that Gajavakra ran what Das described as his "savouries business." His cooking utensils, vessels and the fire place were huddled together in one corner of the room, blackened with soot from the flames, from which "he'd cook, crouched over the fire, from about nine in the morning until about 1:30 pm. Then he'd stop to eat his lunch before loading everything up on to the cart, and leave by around 2 pm." The cart was a cranky, flat-topped wooden construction, sagging under the weight of the savoury snacks it was laden down with. These included *pakodi*—fried onions and curry leaves in a crispy chickpea flour batter—and spicy mixture or *chivda*, a snack comprised of fried puffed rice, nuts and pulses, as well as wide aluminium basins of *masala vada*s and *idli*s, both classic dishes eaten daily across the South of India, prepared from fermented urad dhal. Idlis are steamed, spongy white and circular; vadas, the same shape although often with a hole in the centre, are deep fried and golden brown, and both would have been served with Gajavakra's home-made peanut chutney. The *pakodi*s and mixture would sell first, and then, by around five o'clock, he'd shift to nearer the main market place, picking up trade from men on their way home from work, who would stop to eat idlis and vada. He would stay there, selling from the cart, until everything was gone—sometimes as late as 10 pm—and then he would make his way home, take a bath, eat dinner and sleep. Work would need to begin again at around 6 am the next morning, when he would go to collect firewood and fresh ingredients, take spices and pulses to be ground into flour for batter, and start chopping up vegetables, ready to light the fire again by about 9 am. His mother, meanwhile, would wash up the cooking vessels Gajavakra left behind and help out as and when needed in the kitchen. It was hot, hard work, hunched over a smoky fire, especially in the hot season when temperatures rose to over 40 degrees Celsius in Madras, and for someone with leprosy—whether or not Gajavakra was aware he had it at the time—it would have been harder still.

For Das, however, life remained straightforward. "Look at Anil over the road in his house now," he told me, by way of explanation. I was talking to him outside his current house back in Anandapuram, and he was referring to his neighbour's son. I looked across the road at an eighteen-year-old boy, in red shorts and holey vest, lying sprawled across a string bed. "What's he doing? Nothing. That's what you're like when you're young. I'd just go out and about and play games, that same kind of thing. If I felt like it, I'd maybe go to the shop in the evening, or occasionally I'd be asked to go and get some groceries or take pulses for grinding, but I didn't help out a lot."

Das was also supposed to be studying. Although he originally told me that he had completed his final year school exams in Kumbakonam, as his story unfolded he admitted that he had not actually turned up for those examina-tions. "That's why we'd stayed behind when my father went to Madras," he confessed, "but what can I say? I hadn't prepared for the exam, I didn't feel like doing it, I was lazy. So the family decided I should complete my studies when we got to Madras." Although his attendance at tutorial college in Madras was also patchy—"I was supposed to go every day between 4 pm and 8 pm, but I'd only go two or three times a week"—he did complete the exams this time around, and achieved his secondary school leaving certifi-cate (SSLC), as it was called, in September 1966.

"I just scrapped through," he said. "I managed to pass Hindi without writing anything on the paper at all. In Tamil Nadu, we resented having to learn the language of the north, so I think they used to pass everyone, what-ever they had written. And in the other subjects I got 40s and 50s—nothing special, but enough."

Like many young men in India for whom parents had been unable to secure employment, a period of drifting, maybe a year or two, sometimes more, filled the gap between completing education and getting a job.[2] "I tried to go to some typing classes," he said, "because we thought if I was able to do this I might be able to get a small job in an office somewhere. It was a general idea, someone had suggested it to my father, I think." And Das did go along with it for a while—six days, perhaps—but then stopped. He still knows how to use a keyboard, hammering as heavily on the keys of my laptop computer as he would have done on the old Godrej manual typewriter on which he had been trained, but he never progressed beyond typing with more than two fingers.

The other things he learned around that time were mostly recreational, although some of the skills he developed would serve him well later on. "We played cricket, cards, went to the cinema halls, hung around with street friends and neighbours, Brahmins and non-Brahmins, whoever was around," he told me when I pushed him on how he spent the hours. It was here and at that time he learned to play rummy: "I sat, watching the older men play, worked out the rules, and eventually started joining in." He also picked up a few gambling card games, some of which, like *lappala-bayata* (in Telugu, literally inside-outside, or "over-and-under," as it was usually called in English), still get played by groups of men, huddled relatively discreetly under the trees near the railway line, in Anandapuram at festival times. He explained the rules to me: "It's a simple game: you shuffle the cards, and cut them. I cut a ten, say, and you cut a three. We then deal out the cards, face up, and if a ten comes first, I win. If a three comes first, the hand is yours. It's not a skilled game at all, anyone can play, but it can cost a lot of money. With rummy, you just play for Rs5 or Rs10 per game, not so much."

Although it did not come out in Das's earlier telling of the story—or, indeed, when we fleshed out the details by going over and over the chronology—throw away comments as we walked through his old haunts began to reveal that his own history of absconding from home also started earlier than I had originally thought. As we crossed the bridge that passes over Mambalam station—a stop on the local line not five minutes walk from where they were then living—he remembered the story of how he had been sent by his mother to Madras Central Station to buy a train ticket to Bombay for one of his relatives. As was often the case, he tried to save his own fare by not buying himself a ticket, but this time, unfortunately, the ticket inspectors caught him. "The fine took up half the ticket money," he said, "and as I didn't have enough left to get the ticket I'd been sent out for, I was too afraid to go home. I met up with some of my friends near the railway and I gambled the rest of the money away on cards. Then I just avoided going near the house for a few days, sleeping outside, getting by." Running away or hiding out for a while until potential anger had subsided somewhat, was a remarkably common response to trouble by many of my male informants over the years, and sometimes women too. Although it may not quite have been considered socially acceptable, it was certainly a culturally recognized way of dealing with apparently otherwise irresolvable difficulties. And Gajavakra had already provided Das with a useful template for avoiding head-on domestic collision.[3]

This was not the first time Das had taken off, either. On the bus between Kumbakonam and Chennai—our return journey—he pointed out to me a small town, forty-five minutes out of Kumbakonam, where one of his relatives had once lived. It reminded him of the time that he and his friends had skipped school in Kumbakonam, he reckoned they must have been about fifteen, to go there and see the new Tamil film *Aayirathil Oruvan*—which Das translates as "One in a thousand"—starring M. G. Ramachandran and Jayalalitha, both of whom later became Chief Ministers in Tamil Nadu. I looked up the film some months later, and the dates match: it was released in 1965. "New films used to show here, at that cinema," he said, pointing out of the bus window, "before they reached Kumbakonam, and we could get out here for the 11:45am show, and get back at around the same time school was due to finish, so our families didn't know." Although he claimed to have gone to school most of the time, our discussion also triggered memories of missing classes to play hide and seek in Gandhi Park. Over the years he also spent the occasional night or two sleeping at the bus stand or the station, and once on the school verandah.

It was his knowledge of Mayuram, the town with the cinema, that brought him back there when he wanted to get away from home in Madras a few years later. He had travelled there this time on the train, without a ticket, and had worked for two days in a small tea shop, helping out with washing glasses and pulling water from the well in exchange for food. "Nothing had happened especially, I don't think," he said when I asked him why he had absconded. "I was just interested to see new places, to get away sometimes. It could be boring, being in one place all the time." Perhaps these same sentiments also drove his father.

Back in Madras, Gajavakra was feeling the strain of running his savouries business from home. Subrahmanyam, Parvathi's tax inspector husband, had also expressed concerns that the returns from such a business were scant reward for the effort that had to be exerted, and he encouraged him to attempt something both more ambitious and less physically strenuous. He was also prepared to lend him the money to do it. "'Why do you need to sit in the road from morning to night?' they asked him," according to Das. "They never visited us there, they lived a long way off on the other side of the city, but they heard about the situation one way or another, and wanted to help."

Gajavakra took up his relatives' offer of assistance. In 1967, he rented out a larger building from which to run a meals mess, offering cooked food to students and men working away from home. The family shifted once again—this time to Akhbar Sahib Street, in Triplicane—in order to be close by. We went back to see the mess when we were in Chennai, and although it was smaller than I had imagined from Das's earlier descriptions, it still served the same function for its current occupant. The main part of the building consisted of a deep, narrow room, scarcely wider than the double wooden doors that opened in from the street and extended back maybe 20 or 30 feet. It was dark and cool inside. The diners would have sat, crossed legged, on long mats placed on either side of the floor while servers, balancing great vessels of rice and curries, would have run up and down the space left in the middle, hastily ladling out food on to the leaf plates set before them. Meals, Das remembers, included good quality rice, sambar, rasam, one fried vegetable dish, curd, pickle and, on Sundays, a milk sweet. "Back then we could provide all that for one rupee," Das said. "We had to, because that's what all the other messes did, and we needed to compete. The problem, I think, was that his knowledge of how to organise these things properly was not so good, and that's why things went wrong."

Gajavakra had saved around Rs10,000 from his previous business, and Subrahmanyam had provided another Rs25,000, with which he was able to pay for the lease on the building, buy new cooking vessels and stock up on fuel. "With that backing, he managed to keep things going for a year," Das said, "But then the losses started to stack up again."

Toward the end of Gajavakra's time at the meals hotel, Das also acquired his first job at Ultra Marine Blue, a company that manufactured the blue powder then popular for adding to one's white wash to make it come out blue-white. Subrahmanyam, by now, was a senior tax commissioner, and Ultra Marine Blue fell under his jurisdiction. Das was unsure how the recommendation was actually made, but he suspected his uncle had simply told them that he had a relative, educated up to tenth standard, in need of a job. They would almost certainly have responded favourably to a tax inspector. What Das does remember is that he was summonsed to the factory owner's house, memorable chiefly because it was next door but one to the film star (and later Chief Minister of Andhra Pradesh) N T Rama Rao. "He was a God!" said Das. "Everyday there would be ten or more busloads of people who would come for a glimpse of him. It was before he entered politics, but he played Lord Krishna, and that's how people saw and treated him."

As for the meeting with the boss, Das was left to wait in the hall for some time, and was then called by a servant to meet the big man himself, who sat perched on a wooden swing in the centre of the room. "I told him my uncle had sent me, told him I wanted a job, and he gave me a letter and told me to report to the administration block of the company next morning."

"It was a big factory, in Ambattur," Das recalled. "I think probably more than one thousand people worked there. There were different blocks for mixing and grinding and this and that, but I never went onto the factory floor, only into the office section." Ambattur is an industrial area on the north-west periphery of Madras, eleven miles from where Das's family were living in Triplicane, and it took him around an hour to get there each morning on the local train for an 8am start.

"I wasn't doing accounts work then," Das said, "but I think the plan for the future might have been that. To start with, in that first month, I was just expected to collect together paperwork, do the filing, that kind of thing. Someone would say, come here, take this dossier over there to the man on that desk, and I'd simply do it. No shouting or unpleasantness, just 'Oh, Mohandas! Come here, take this over there!,' like that."

It was, by his own account, relatively easy work, but it was also clear from Das's depiction that the work held no particular interest. "It was all right, actually," he told me, "but did I enjoy it? What was there to like or not to like? It was just a job, that's all. I didn't think much about it." He did dislike settling into the routine though. "Every morning it would be out of bed by 5 am to take a bath and get ready, and then trying to get on the full train during the busiest time, and a thirty minute walk to the factory once I got off at the station. And there was no proper food, only what I took with me in my tiffin box."

The job lasted a month, if that. Das could not even recall ever having drawn a salary. "I was young, it wasn't the time for working," he shrugged. Then he went on to explain how, one morning, he had been running late, had missed the usual train, and was worried that he would be reprimanded for his tardiness. "So I stayed away that day, I had a few rupees in my pocket from the house, and I ran into another friend, so we went off to the cinema. Later we found some more friends and sat around and played cards until it would have been time to return home, and at the usual time I went back to the house."

"The next day, I suppose I felt nervous about having not been in the day before, so I skipped work again, and did the same sort of thing as I did before. And then I carried on like that for three or four days, returning to the house at the right time. Somehow my mother found out, and then there was a row."

His mother was uncharacteristically angry. "I told her that I didn't want to go there any more, that I didn't like the job, and she shouted, said that my uncle had recommended me, that I would spoil his good name and that it wasn't right. So I took some money and left the house, absconded."

With nothing more than the cash he had in his pocket and the clothes he was wearing, Das took off to Madras Central Railway Station, and boarded a train that took him 1,000 miles up along the coast to Howrah, across the Howrah bridge from Calcutta in West Bengal. From there, calmer now but not in a mood to return home and enjoying the sense of freedom, he randomly boarded another train, finally ending up in Barara, in Haryana. Not much interested in what he found there, he travelled back to Calcutta, and this time got talking to a fellow Tamilian boy on the train. His new friend told him that he worked for a group of money-lenders and debt collectors from Tamil Nadu who were operating in Calcutta, cycling around and collecting money on their behalf. It was, he told Das, straightforward work: he was reasonably well paid and the group looked after him. "'Come with me!' he said," Das recalled, "'I'll recommend you, and we can work together!' So I thought, okay, why not? I don't have any money and I need to get by, so I'll give it a try."

"He took me to meet them, the money lenders, nearby the station, and they said, all right, you can help out with cooking, fetching water, cleaning out the cooking vessels and that kind of thing, and we'll feed you and take care of you. I agreed, but in the end I only stayed for a day or two, the work wasn't suitable for me, and I didn't want to stay. I'd had no idea what to do, actually, which is why I ended up there. I just got on a train without thinking anything very much and went. I suppose I thought I'd go to Calcutta and get a job . . . but I felt, when I got there, it was too far away from home, what could I do there? After leaving those debt collecting people I went to the bridge to sleep and, when I woke up, I went and got on another train, back to Madras."

Although Das returned to his family's city, however, he did not return home. He was not certain, when he arrived at the station, what to do. There is an area to the left as you come out of Madras Central station, where the old cycle rickshaws tout for business and unofficial traders hawk their goods to the passing hordes of people as they come in and out of the station. Das found a place there to sit quietly on the raised pavement, between a pan and tobacco stall and a fruit seller. It was the fruit seller, Syamala, who spotted him there and asked him who he was and where he had come from. "I told her I was a Brahmin boy and gave her the name of my native place," said Das, "but I didn't tell her my family was now living in Madras. I said I'd had a fight with my mother and father back in my village, that they'd beaten me and so I'd run away. I needed to give her some kind of reason, no? She'd asked the question, so I had to tell her something."

Syamala had nodded sympathetically. "Okay," she said, "You sit here for a while, and watch my stall for me. I'll be back in ten minutes." So Das did. There were not many customers in that time, but when they came he took the money for the bananas they bought and put it in the bag Syamala had left him with. It was a simple, makeshift stall, less sophisticated even than his father's trolley across the city in Mamballam had been: just a small wooden pallet, enlarged with a thin sheet of wood that, covered with old newspapers, made a platform for the bananas. A pile of newspapers to one side, along with a ball of string and a razor blade to cut it with, provided packaging; a small shopping bag containing her lunch in a steel tiffin carrier and a brass pot filled with drinking water on the other side offered everything else she needed to keep trading. Das sat in the centre. "I didn't know it then," he explained, "but she was sitting watching me from somewhere on the other side of the road, looking out to see if I pocketed the money I took for myself or ate her bananas. And she saw that I didn't, that I took ten or twenty rupees business from passers-by, that I wasn't cheating her. So when she came back, she said to me, 'All right, I can see you're a good Brahmin boy, if you like you can stay here at the roadside with us and help on the stall sometimes, and we'll help you in return.' So that was what happened."

Das would sleep on the wide pavement that ran down the side of the station and which was protected from the road by the market stalls that had illegally set up in front of it. Every now and then, he would mind Syamala's fruit stall for her. "If I sat there for a while she'd provide some tiffin and some tea, and occasionally some money, just two or three rupees once in a while, and it was enough. Back then, I was young, I was a good Brahmin boy who had come straight from my family home, so I didn't have too many bad habits. I didn't smoke or drink or go with prostitutes or other things, so I didn't have much expenditure to bear." It was also a relatively safe place to stay, alongside the other traders, station porters and rickshaw wallahs, with large trees providing shade and the station wall offering additional protection from the elements.

It was easy to immerse oneself in station life. "So many people live there, other young people like me, too, who I got to know and played cards and other things with. I didn't stand out too much. If there were police around, I'd stay close by Syamala on the fruit stall, otherwise sometimes I'd go inside the station and—learning what to do from those around me—would ask people if they wanted help carrying their luggage, and they'd give me a few paise too. We were very free."

Occasionally there was trouble. "Sometimes, because we weren't registered porters, the railway police would be standing there waiting for us out of sight near the entrance, and as we came out they would pounce. They'd take the luggage we were carrying away from us and give it to another porter, and then they'd take us to their room inside the railway station for a few hours. We'd wait there, take a beating, and then, most of the time, get sent away. Sometimes they'd keep us there for longer, make a case and issue a fine. If they did that, Syamala would come and bail me out, pay them a bribe or the fine. These days the fine is around Rs1,500, but back then it wasn't so much."

Why, I asked him, was Syamala so ready to help him out? What was in it for her? Das shrugged. Perhaps I am too cynical. "Only that she had someone reliable to mind her stall and her things," he guessed. "I was just a boy, she was more than forty, and sometimes she and her husband would also call me to go to their house for food. They weren't Brahmins, they were very low caste, and I think they had respect and trust for me because I was a Brahmin boy: I was very fair skinned back in those days, I looked good, so they knew I wasn't some kind of rowdy. And I was useful to have around: when she wanted some idlis or some tea, she could give me a few rupees and I'd go and collect them for her; when she needed to be somewhere else I could mind her things, sell her fruit."

By his own reckoning, Das spent around three or four months on the station that year. He might well have stayed there longer, too, had someone who knew his family not spotted him. "They heard from someone that I was there, and my father, I think it was, came for me. When I saw him, I turned away to hide, but he'd already spotted me and called out my name, and I thought, well, I'm tired already of living like this, perhaps I should just go home now, there's a chance there of a different kind of life. So I went back with him. And my mother, she wasn't still angry by then, she was just pleased to see me."

It was 1968 and, for the next few months, life fell back into the old routines: "This and that, time passing, looking around for some work . . . I was still just a boy." His father worked at the meals mess all day, his mother kept house, and his younger brother attended school. But then an opportunity arose for Das to go to Bombay, and, although he was not aware it would be many years before he saw any of his family members again, Das left his home in Madras for the very last time.

NOTES

1. For an anthropological overview of everyday Hinduism, see C. J. Fuller, *The Camphor Flame: Popular Hinduism and Society in India* (Princeton: Princeton University Press, 2004) and Kim Knott, *Hinduism: A Very Short Introduction* (Oxford: Oxford University Press, 1998).

2. This phenomenon, picked up elsewhere in the literature, is the specific focus of Craig Jeffrey's "Timepass: Youth, Class, and time among unemployed young men in India," *American Ethnologist*, 7, 3 (2010a): 465–481; and his monograph *Timepass: Youth, Class, and the Politics of Waiting in India* (Stanford: Stanford University Press, 2010b).

3. Although, as far as I know, there have no specific ethnographic studies of this apparent tendency toward flight among men (and occasionally women) from lower socio-conomic groups in India, the regularity of its occurrence among my own informants over the years did suggest that this was not just a case of random acts but a social phenomenon. It also resonated, for me, with the historical account of fugue in eighteenth century France provided by the philosopher Ian Hacking, *Mad Travelers: Reflections on the reality of transient mental illnesses* (Cambridge, Mass: Harvard University Press, 1998).

Chapter Three

Bombay

After his adventures on Madras Central Station, Das's family was keen that he should be occupied with a job as soon as possible. It was Subrahmanyam who came to the rescue, presumably at the behest of Das's mother, although he too might have had a vested interest in keeping his wife's relatives off the street. Apart from the social embarrassment it could have caused to someone of his social standing, Subrahmanyam was, by Das's own account, a man with a strong sense of responsibility. "He was strict and religious," Das said, "and he had faith as a Hindu in God. He wasn't the kind of tax inspector who would exempt someone from a payment if they paid him a bribe. Maybe he'd accept a gift—a basket of mangoes, say—but even that I don't know for sure. My faith is that he wouldn't demand money or other favours from people, even though they would be well disposed towards him when he mentioned he had relatives who needed jobs! I had respect, not fear, for him."

Das did not see Subrahmanyam again after he returned home from the station, which saved his own embarrassment. It was not long though before he received a message telling him about an opportunity in Bombay, where Subrahmanyam and Parvathi were now stationed, along with a letter to produce for the employer when he got there. Within days he had packed his case—his school-leaving certificate included—and purchased, as he remembers vividly, a Rs32 one-way ticket to the opposite side of the country. His mother cautioned him to work hard, to take care of his health and to eat properly. Then he left the family home for the last time. It was late 1968.

Das's departure marked something of a mass exodus from the family home in Madras. A couple of months later, at the behest of Parvathi, his mother also travelled to Bombay, to help her run the family following the birth of their third child, Suresh. Parvathi is often described, in accounts both from Das and his brother Chandra Prakash, either as a patient or as someone who suffered "weakness." "She might have had asthma, I think," Das once told me, vaguely, but asthma was a term often attributed to women who suffered from a generalized kind of poorliness and needed external help. The fact that they could summons such help was also an indication of their relative social status. In any case, it was common for women to travel often long distances to stay with female kin during their pregnancies and deliveries, and so there was nothing especially unusual about Subbalakshmi's visit to Bombay. The plan was that she should stay for two or three months and then return to her husband and youngest son in Madras.

Within days of her departure, however, Gajavakra took the opportunity to escape his canteen's mounting debts. He could no longer pay the rice man or the vegetable sellers, the rent was in arrears, and his credit had run out. Running a business, Das conceded, was not his father's strongest point. Before he left, Gajavakra delivered Chandra Prakash, then aged eight, into the care of the eldest of his three younger brothers, who was living in Trichy. "When my mother first went to Bombay," Chandra Prakash told me, "the family decided I should stay with my father in Madras so I didn't interrupt my schooling any more. I was about to start third class." When Gajavakra also left, his brother, a Tamil Pandit and therefore well-versed in Hindu scripture and religious practices, was considered the most suitable guardian.

Das was, he recalled vaguely, aware of his mother's presence in Bombay, even though he never visited her during his years there. He thinks he must also have received word, probably by letter sometime later, about his father's departure, although he was hazy on the details of what happened to his brother, and was as interested as I was when I interviewed Chandra Prakash about his own movements in hearing the details.

Bombay was a much bigger, more cosmopolitan city than Madras, but although Das had never been there before, it held little fear for him. "I didn't know the language, so I wondered how I would get by without Marathi or Hindi, but no, otherwise I wasn't afraid. I'd already spent time wandering, going here and there and sleeping for days on end in the street, so going away for a job, knowing I had a room to stay in and a place to keep my things at the workplace, that was no problem for me!"

The job, this time, was at a company called the Simac Group of India Limited, which assembled knitting machines. The factory was in the suburb of Goregaon, where Das went to meet the owner and his family. The stores, where he was to live and work, were eight miles south in Santa Cruz, on the corner of what is now a busy intersection. Back then, it was still a relatively quiet suburb. "I directly met the boss first," he remembered. "Somebody offered me a seat and I waited for a while until he arrived, and he suddenly appeared, smiled and said, 'Ahh! So you're the boy!' He introduced me to his two sons who, in turn, treated me like their own adopted son. I was given a lot of freedom to go here and there around the workplace and to fit in where

I wanted." There were around one hundred employees in total, although only thirty in Santa Cruz, where Das's official designation was as a storekeeper.

"I was young and happy," Das told me, exuding an enthusiasm, as he recalled his time there, which suggested his role was more fulfilling than the work he had done at Ultra Marine Blue. The freedom offered by living away from home no doubt also played a part. "There were two brothers from Uttar Pradesh who worked in the store with me," he said, "called Rama and Seth Mishra. Rama Mishra was the watchman, and the other one was a worker, and like me they both slept in the building at night. I didn't know their language, they spoke Hindi, but with English and the words I started to pick up we got by, and I'd enjoy sitting and chatting and laughing with them. They'd cook northern Indian food for themselves sometimes too, which they'd share with me. It was all new to me—we didn't have that kind of cooking in Madras. They'd make dry chapattis and we'd eat them with a very spicy potato curry. Happy times!"

Das's working hours, he remembers with his typical precision for numbers, were from 8am to 1pm, and from 2pm to 5pm, Monday to Saturday. "My job was issuing the materials out from the stores—screws, plates, that kind of thing—and in between times I could go around the place and sit in different places if I got bored. I was independent, so I learned how to make up one of the machines too. It wasn't necessary, that wasn't my job, but it made things more interesting. I felt like one of the bosses there! Like a factory owner! Even the sons of the owner, when they came down to Santa Cruz, they'd come in and call me over to share coffee, drinks, sweets, things like that. They didn't do that with the other staff, but with me, they always did."

Caste might have had something to do with Das's special treatment, but it also had something to do with his connections. "I was the person who had been recommended by the Income Tax Commissioner, no?!" he laughed, "So I think they didn't want to give me anything to complain about!" Subrahman-yam had been posted to Bombay and was living in Chembur with Parvathi and their children. The factory would have come under his jurisdiction. He was also at the most senior post of his career: he spent the next decade in Bombay, right up until his retirement. Das did not visit Chembur though, despite it being only five or six miles from Santa Cruz, and his mother also living there. "After everything that had happened before, with me leaving the last job and him doing so much for me," he said, "I felt too embarrassed to face him. It was best to leave them there and get on with things."

Das was not, in any case, lonely. The Mishra brothers introduced him early on to a Tamil family. The wife, Ponnamma, worked in the factory and they lived just opposite the factory gates. He visited their house a few times and ate with them whenever Ponnamma prepared Tamil specialities, as she did at festival times. Such southern delicacies, not commonplace in the area at that time, kept alive memories of home. Links to regional identities, in this city of migrants, were important: eating southern and, more particularly, Tamil vegetarian food, helped to constitute Das to himself as what he was.

Food, whether eaten at the homes of his fellow workers or purchased locally, was in any case generally good. There was a café opposite the workplace where he would buy potato *vada* (a spicy potato patty served in a white bun) or *usal* (bean sprouts in a spicy sauce) for his breakfast, and rice or chapatti and Maharashtrian curries for his lunch. "If I had a bit of cash I might also go somewhere for tandoori food," he said, licking his lips at the thought. "Channa masala, tandoor roti, mattar paneer . . . it was all new, tasty food for me, and I liked it."

He also made friends with some of the other workers, including a Roman Catholic called Edgar Popham, who took him home to meet his family. "He was a very tall man, about forty or forty-five years old, and he lived with his wife and their child, very close to the factory. They sold *arrack* [a fermented home brew], and he liked to drink it, too! But I never took alcohol, not back in those days. Good Brahmin boys didn't take liquor. I'd just go and sit there with them, eat some mixture or some biscuits, just time passing."

Gurinder, another worker, had come to Bombay from the Punjab, and was enjoying an affair with a local married woman. "He took me with him to her house once, for some *bhang*—you know that drink? They grind together cannabis leaves and buds and mix it with milk, sugar and some spices. It was very common in Bombay. You drink it and it makes you laugh and laugh! The time we went to Gurinder's girlfriend's house to drink some was on a special day—Baisakhi, I think it must have been, the Punjabi harvest festival—because *bhang* was the thing to drink during that celebration. I can remember the laughter."

Das went on: "That woman's husband was also there, but I don't think he minded too much about Gurinder and his wife. He was old and very weak and she was very young, so as long as she fed him and looked after him he wasn't really bothered. Of course, Gurinder didn't fondle her or anything in front of the husband! They were just talking and that, but he knew, all the same, and it was okay."

In addition to hanging out at colleagues' houses during leave and festival periods, Das got to know the immediate surrounding area fairly well. Juhu beach was only a short bus ride away, and he found it pleasant to go and sit there, eat some Bombay street food and look out across the water, in his free time. On one occasion, he ran into another of his work colleagues, a fitter called Ashok, who was on his way to the infamous Grant Road, and expressed surprise that Das had never been there. "'You've never heard of it?!' he said to me, 'I thought everyone knew about Grant Road. Come with me, I'll take you there for a look.'"

"So he took me there with him on the bus and the local train—it must have taken an hour or so to get there—and then I saw them, all these women, standing out there in front of the houses. I was shocked: how is this acceptable, I thought, women dressed like this? I didn't understand, not straight away, what was going on here. They were standing there wearing nothing but petticoats and small bodices on their top halves. They'd have a few accessories on, too, necklaces and bangles, earrings, that kind of thing. Lots of them wore make-up, as well."

The women were, to Das's untrained eyes, the antithesis of everything he had been brought up to see as normative femininity.[1] Instead of saris protecting their modesty they revealed more flesh than he had ever seen; instead of hair neatly plaited and tied back their thick black tresses hung loose and carefree around their shoulders; and instead of discreet jewelry and no make-up other than a smudge of vermillion powder on their temples to mark their married status, these women boasted big, brash ornaments, bright nail polish and red lipstick. He had, quite literally, never seen anything like them before.

These women, as Ashok explained to him, were working as prostitutes, and Grant Road was, and still is, a red light area. "Back in those days though, it was a higher-class kind of place than it is now," Das told me. "Back then, you'd get doctors, policemen, all kinds of people going there. Now it's more of a working men's kind of place." On that visit, Das and Ashok were just there to watch, taking in the spectacle for a while before going on to the cinema. "And that's what we started doing on Sundays, when we had time off. We'd go over to Grant Road, take a walk down the road and have a look at all the women, observe how men would approach them, and then we'd watch a movie, get something to eat, and finally go back to Santa Cruz."

After several months of getting to know the area, however, Das decided to visit Grant Road on his own. "I'd been hearing them call out to us every week, 'Hey! Over here, ten bucks, ten bucks!' So I thought, okay, why not? I have ten bucks, I'll go inside and see what it's like. And that was my first experience of sex. When I got in the building, there were separate rooms and everything, and there were six girls in there: 'Just come in and choose who you like the look of!' they said to me outside, so I just looked up quickly, thought the first one I saw looked all right, so I pointed and said, 'yes, she's okay!' I knew nothing at the time. I was shy, but they were the experts, they did everything for me. And afterwards, it felt good. I felt that I was a man, not a boy any more. A woman had accepted me as a man, and so I also felt very happy about it."

Das visited the place alone several times after that in the years that followed, becoming more of a connoisseur as his experience grew. "One time I'd go and think, hmm, today I'll choose a Nepalese girl, see what she is like, and another time I might want to experience a Tamil girl. We can try different things, no? And the great thing about Nepalese girls, even though they were often more expensive, is that they'd never steal from you. That was my experience. Even if you take your trousers off and leave your wallet in them on the bed, they'll not try to take it. They might just ask for Rs50 *baksheesh* as well as the fee, that's all, just some extra money that the pimp or whoever can't take from them. In other places, with some of the other women, it's different. They'll tell you to hang your clothes on a peg and then, when you're engaged in sex, they'll give a signal to another girl who will slip into the room and take your money. It's possible because your concentration is elsewhere at those moments, no?"

"It happened to me once. They took Rs1,000—all the money I had, and it was a lot in those days. I didn't realize until after I'd left, and then I went back and asked them, did you take my money? They turned very fierce when I asked that. Four or five more of them seemed to appear from nowhere, and I was surrounded. 'What are you accusing us of?!' they shouted at me, and then all of them grabbed at me and started beating me. I yelled out that I'd call the police on them and they laughed. One of them turned away and threw the money down on the bed. 'You see that? There's your money, why did you try to say we'd taken it?!' she said, 'you must have left it there.' I grabbed it up and got out of there quickly. They were like a group of devils, the way they had come towards me like that!"

The attack did not put Das off subsequent sexual encounters, but it did teach him to be more careful. When he visited Grant Road in future he took only the money he needed along with him.

His visits were curtailed for a while, however, by other events that took shape around eight months after his arrival in Bombay. They were provoked by something small: a thickening of one of his earlobes, to be precise, and a small patch there of paler skin, with no feeling. It was the watchman, Rama Mishra, who first noticed it, pointed it out and told Das he ought to see a doctor about it. When he did, the doctor did not say much, except to tell him he needed some more checks at a specialist hospital, and jotted down details of how to find the hospital he needed to attend in Wadala, about six miles away. "I didn't know what kind of hospital it was until I got there," Das remembers, "and then I got there and I saw the signs outside, saying it was a leprosy hospital. It was a shock. I thought, 'Oh my God! I've got this terrible disease.' I thought it was all over for me. And right there, at that moment, even before I went in, I made the decision that I wouldn't go back to the store room in Santa Cruz."

"I didn't really know anything about leprosy in those days," he said. "I hadn't seen real patients, close-up, but I'd seen actors dressed up as lepers in films at the cinema, and I thought, oh my God! My hands will go! My fingers will drop off! My life is gone! But I still went in anyway. They took some blood, did some kind of tests, and told me to come back for the results the next day. I slept outside on the pavement, and when I went back they said that the test had come out as six-plus—that meant I was full of leprosy—and that I needed to take treatment, Dapsone tablets, for a couple of years."

"What could I have done?" he went on. "I didn't want to go to my uncle's place. My mother was with them by then, and Subrahmanyam and Parvathi also had three children of their own, who my mother was helping to look after. So I thought to myself, why should I unnecessarily bring another burden on them? They were caring for my mother, and they had recommended me for a job. That was enough, I think."[2]

Besides, domestic family life in a Bombay suburb held no particular attraction: Das was now used to being free to do what he wanted, and was also well versed in getting by living on the streets. "This wasn't the first time I'd lived on the pavement," as Das put it, "I'd spent that time on Madras Central Station, and I'd travelled to Calcutta and other places on my own, so it was a life I knew. And the reason I went from the hospital directly to the train station is that I knew, once I'd been told I had leprosy, that I couldn't do other kinds of work. I wouldn't be able to work in a meals hotel or a tea stand, for example: people wouldn't accept those things from me if they knew I had leprosy. And I don't think people would have accepted me back at Simac, either. I was, I thought at the time, only suitable for carrying luggage for tips, wandering here and there. So when I got to the station, I just stayed there."

In shorter versions of Das's life story, this particular event was recounted as the initial rupture in what had otherwise been a straightforward life trajectory. In such renderings of his story, the dramatic quality of his departure—from a promising career to a life on the streets—attests to the socially devastating quality of leprosy. The stigma and sense of shame associated with it was so strong, the story implies, that victims of the disease felt compelled to abandon their homes and their families. Certainly, there is a ring of truth to this, and it would be wrong to under-estimate the socially transformative effects of diseases, which, especially in the case of leprosy, are so saturated in historical and culturally specific meanings. But in Das's case, and for many of the others I encountered in my work with people affected by leprosy, the disease was just one, albeit important, factor in how things turned out. Das's father, Gajavakra, had already provided a well-defined template for male flight as a response to seemingly intractable problems, one that was refined throughout Das's formative years with each subsequent departure from the family home. Das, too, was accustomed by now to absconding: it was a proven way of circumventing whatever problems he had faced, and also offered new and exciting alternatives to a dull *status quo*. I accept Das's insistence that his discovery of leprosy was the immediate trigger for his departure from Simac, but I also suspect that, sooner or later, Das would have moved on anyway.

As it was, Das did not even return to Santa Cruz for his suitcase and his things. The factory owners, Das discovered years later, "made a big drama out of it. Maybe they were afraid of what Subrahmanyam would do when he found out, or maybe the watchman, Rama Mishra, blamed me for some pilfering that he had done. But they told my family I had stolen some money and other items and run off. It was a way of protecting themselves. My uncle asked them what had happened, told them he'd repay them whatever I had taken, but they said, 'oh no sir! That's not necessary. No problem sir!' I discovered all this after a very long time. But the truth was that I left with nothing at all, just the clothes I was wearing."

He never met Subrahmanyam again, although he did spot him once, catching a train from the station, and successfully hid. He also ran into Edgar Popham one day, a few years later. He was no longer working in the factory, but driving a taxi. "I saw him outside the station, and we greeted each other cordially, said hello and exchanged pleasantries, but that's about all," said Das. "He was still running the arrack business on the side, I think."

It was late 1969 or early 1970, Das was nineteen years old, and although he had never been someone to think too much about the future, the things that he had taken for granted would happen one day, like marriage and children, no longer seemed a possibility. "That's why I only took the drugs they had given me at the hospital for a few days, and then I threw them out. What was the point? If I took them I wasn't going to be cured tomorrow, the next day, or even the next year. My understanding then was that once leprosy comes, it can't really be treated. So I neglected myself."

Day-to-day life, however, was initially not so much different on Dadar station, his new home, to the life he had lived on Madras Central. "We changed our clothes once or twice a week, slept on the raised pavements, went into the trains to wash our hands and faces, slept and ate when we could." Most days, having slept for a few hours on a couple of mats or some layers of cardboard on the station platform, Das and his fellow unofficial porters would rise early, at around 4:30am, when the first train of the morning came in: the 4:45am passenger from Ahmedabad. "We'd freshen up a bit, use the facilities on the train to wash, and would take a tea from one of the *chai wallahs* on the station," Das remembered. "Then we'd wait for a train to come, and try to get work carrying the luggage when the passengers got off. Up until around 8:30am it would be very busy, there were maybe six or seven trains in before then, including a long distance one to Viramgam in Gujarat. We'd try to reserve seats for passengers on that one, leaping on to the train before anyone else could and sitting there until the passengers found us."

Finding accommodation for incoming passengers was another source of income. "Sometimes people would ask us to find them hotels, and so we'd take them to somewhere we knew. They'd give us maybe Rs10, and we could also take more from the hotel in commission, making Rs40 or Rs50 a time in total. Some hotels readily paid commission, some didn't. And it didn't take us long to work out which ones were the best for us, and those were the ones we'd take the passengers to. Even if they were a bit far from the station, we'd convince them that they would be the best places to stay. If they said, 'but isn't there somewhere closer?' or 'what about those hotels over there?,' we'd just tell them, 'No, no, they are full sir,' and 'the place I'm taking you to, that is so much better, cheapest and best sir! Very good hotel sir, just a little bit further from here . . . come on sir!' And if we took two or three passengers at the same time, we'd get commission for each one. If the hotels gave us money, we'd go back, if they refused, next time we wouldn't bother. And often they'd give out their cards too, to encourage us to come back: Hotel Mother India, Hotel Royal Guest House . . . there were quite a few places that we could take people to!"

Once the train to Viramgam had left the station, Das would take some breakfast in the station canteen: bread or chapatti, or sometimes puri or usal, eaten with the usual chutneys or potato curry. "After that, at around 10am, we'd usually start playing cards with the other people living on the station, in a fairly discreet place so that we could gamble." Das showed me the location when we visited during the monsoon in 2011. They would sit under the shadows cast by Tilak Bridge, just behind the station and a shelter for many who lived on the streets, or on the green space, now built up, that stretched out from it. "Gambling was just a way of passing the time," Das said. "If we were playing rummy and it felt that it was going too slowly, we'd speed things up a bit with some faster games." This would continue for a couple of hours, until around noon, and then they'd go and eat—rice and dhal or *vada pav*, which Bombay was famous for—before finding a place to rest through the hottest part of the day. "We'd sleep overhead on the platform roof, sometimes, or under the bridge, because it was shady there. And at about 4pm we'd wake up, and start over again: I'd wash my face, go and have a tea, and get set up for when the trains started going again at around 6pm, mostly the trains going out of Bombay. And we'd do our work finding places for the passengers to sit or carrying their bags for them." It was not easy getting accepted by the others who lived and worked on the station. New porters were a threat to their already precarious livelihoods. The trick, as Das explained it, was to lie low and to befriend someone who was already established: in his case, a fellow Tamilian, who ran one of the station's card schools. "Being away, far from home, Tamilians are always drawn together," he said, "ready to look out for one another. And gradually, as time goes on, you become a known face, someone who can be trusted." He also made sure he kept on the right side of Reuben, the chief porter, by handing over a hefty cut of every transaction he made.

On a more personal level, keeping clean was one of the biggest challenges of living on the station, but Das learned quickly from those around him and drew on his experience from Madras. There were nearby markets selling cheap, second hand clothes, and—although some people laundered them—it was common to wear them until they were dirty and then discard them in favour of replacements. For bathing, in addition to using the piped water in the toilet cubicles on the long distance trains, Das would occasionally travel to Bandara: "There was a big pipeline in the wasteland there, but it leaked quite badly, and so there was a flow of good, clean water. We'd bath in it and wash our clothes sometimes." There was also a barber's shop near Dadar station which, in addition to offering haircuts and wet shaves, also had some cubicles at the back for bathing in. "He'd take Rs2 or 3," Das recalled, "and for that he'd provide a bucket of hot water, soap and a towel. There were three or four bathrooms at the back of the shop, in the courtyard. You had to go out of the station for that, though. Inside the station there was only the waiting hall, but if we got caught using those facilities we'd be beaten and thrown out. There was the yard where they hosed down the trains, and sometimes we'd go there, so there were plenty of opportunities if we looked out for them."

Toward the end of his second year on the station, however—sometime in 1971—Das started to become, in his own words, "very weak." He had fevers and leg pains, wanted to sleep all the time and found it difficult to walk. Luckily for him, he had struck up friendships with several others who worked on the station, including Gopi, another fellow Tamilian, who had arrived after Das. "There were a few porters who were unhappy about him being there," Das said, "so I helped him in the same way that others had helped me. I shared my food with him, invited him to play cards with us, and showed him how to get seats for passengers." Later on, Gopi ended up making most of his money as a ticket tout on one of the other Bombay stations, buying up tickets for the Bombay to Delhi Rajdhani train and selling them on the black market, at highly inflated prices, to those unable to get reservations. He eventually built the business up into a travel agency, rented his own office and built himself a house, but when Das first knew him, in the early 1970s, he lived on the station. Gopi recognized Das's symptoms—he had a friend who had also had leprosy—and he knew about a hospital in Gujarat where that friend was getting treatment. "He packed me off there on the train with one of his friends to accompany me," Das said, "and even sent me spending money when I was there. I stayed for six months in the end. I felt so weak at first I could hardly walk, and I was very dizzy. Once I'd been admitted I took full rest."

Compared to his recollections of time on the station, Das's memories of the hospital remain fairly fuzzy, probably because he was unwell at the time and in rest mode rather than in a state of permanent alert to ensure his daily survival. "The method for giving us food," he said, "was that even if you were in bed on the ward, when they rang this bell you had to get up and go to the canteen and collect your ration: usually some chapattis and some curries. Then we'd come back, after food, and wait for the next meal. They'd ring the bell, and off we'd go again. Sometimes it would ring at other times, too—not every day, but if they'd been a visit from, say, some Marwaris [business people] to donate their excess provisions or clothes, we'd be called to receive those things too. People liked to bring sweets, fruit, things like that, as gifts for the leprosy affected." Such gifting, as I had also observed, many years later, in schools for disabled children and in urban begging settlements, was commonplace across India; a way for benefactors to acquire spiritual merit and offset their sins. It also helped to keep the excluded in their place.[3]

The hospital was, Das thought, run by the Government rather than missionaries, and was situated on the outskirts of the local town, with a leprosy colony—for the long-stay patients—adjoining it. Das did not get to know the area very well, however, because patients were, at least officially, confined to their wards: "After you'd been there a while, and if you became friendly with the gateman, then you could go outside every now and then, but mostly we'd hang around the compound." Das was only twenty at the time, and one of the youngest members of the ward, but despite the relatively humdrum routine he stayed put, taking his medication, for the next six months. The new multi-drug therapy had just become available. "It was boring but okay," he recalled. "I liked to read books to pass the time, and although I couldn't identify the individual characters in Hindi script—which most of the books we had access to were written in—I managed to make out whole words. And because I had a lot of time on my hands, I learnt to read basic Hindi over that period." Other patients were from nearer the local area.

Otherwise, life was constituted by a daily routine of receiving medicine from the ward boy, taking tea, bathing, eating and taking rest. It was, by his own account, what he needed at the time, but once he started to feel better Das became restless again. Rigid routine was always something Das had rallied against. "I noticed one day that the watchman wasn't there on the gate," he said, "so I just strolled out, went to the station and took the train to Bombay." Gopi had shifted his business to Bombay Central by then, but Das, who had four or five other friends still on Dadar Station, went back to the location he knew.

"I carried on as before," he said, "finding people seats on trains, taking them to hotels and carrying their luggage for them. And we also played a lot of rummy in between times, and 'in-and-out,' which was the popular game for playing at stations, because it was fast and you could finish a game quickly if the police or other authorities turned up. Then, one of the card school organizers, the Tamil man who had looked after me when I first arrived at the station, needed to go away for while, so he handed over responsibility for the cards to me."

In response to my question about what that entailed he told me: "As the organizer, you provide the mats that we all sit on and the packs of cards. Then you get everyone together, the other porters who want to play, and take some money from them to join in. If you see the police coming, you either pack everything up and move things on, or you pay them something to leave us alone. If there weren't enough players, I'd join in myself. And doing that, for a whole night, you could sometimes make a lot of money, even after paying off the police. It wouldn't happen every night, maybe two or three times a week. And some of the money would go on sending the railway boys—the younger boys who slept and begged on the station—off to get coffee and snacks for us, some would go on new packs of cards, and so on. It was just a side thing, something I did in between carrying luggage. I did it for about two years, from 1972 to 1974."

It was also while he was living on Dadar station that Das made his one concession to what had otherwise been a strict Brahmin vegetarian diet. "Sometimes, when you were on the station, the only thing available on the food carts would be omelette and bread, so I started to take it. The first time I had egg, it was mixed with tomatoes and spices, so it didn't feel as though I was really eating anything different to usual, and I got used to it. But I never took boiled egg, or egg curry made with whole boiled eggs. And I don't like to take too many omelettes either, but that mixture of egg and tomato with carom [chilli powder], that was good and tasty. I never took mutton though, not once. If only meat was available, I would just make do with bread and special tea." Otherwise he ate much as he had done elsewhere in Bombay: chapatti or bread for breakfast, chapatti or rice for lunch, and outside food, from tandoori roast curries to "full meals"—curries with curd and pickles, accompanied by large quantities of rice—in the evenings.

Other than food and occasional changes of clothes, there was not much other essential expenditure for a single man living and working on a Bombay railway station platform. But despite a relatively high income from portering, the card school and commissions from hotels, Das never saved. "What was the point? I had leprosy and that was that: I wasn't going to get married, have children. I was just getting by, day-to-day, until I died. If I made Rs1,000 one day, I'd get through Rs1,000. That's how it was."

In addition to using up his money gambling at cards—"I'd often just keep on going until there was nothing left. Then you'd go to sleep with your pockets empty, and get up and start earning all over again the next morning"—Bombay was an easy place to get through money in the 1970s. "In those days," as Das recalled, "we had the Matka, or the numbers, in Bombay. There was lots of excitement around it at the time." The man who pioneered it—Ratan Kathri, or the "Matka King," as he was known—would draw the first numbers from a new pack of cards at 9pm every evening. "So if he drew, say, a two, a four and a five, you could win something if you had the last digit of the sum of those numbers," Das explained it to me—several times, because his mathematics is much sharper than mine. 'In that case, you'd add two, four and five, which makes eleven, so the extra number would be one, yes? If you'd put a bet of twenty-five paise on that number, the lowest bet, you stood to win Rs2.25. For a rupee stake you could make Rs9."

"Then, at 12 o'clock, you'd get the second numbers, drawn in the same way. And you could place bets anywhere: the bookies would have these notebooks with carbon paper slips, they'd write your number on the slip for you, tear it off and take your bet. The odds were good, with that system. I think that later on, the Government took everything from that man, Ratan Kathri. I once saw him, just a few years ago, when someone pointed him out to me in Bombay, and he looked like a pauper. But there was a lot of money around in the *Matka* back then."[4]

Grant Road was another outlet for disposing of excess money, although Das claims his visits there were infrequent once he knew he had leprosy. Initially, he said he was worried that he might pass on his condition to the women he had sex with, but later he admitted that he was more afraid of rejection. "I thought, if I go inside those houses, maybe they'd spot the signs and tell me to go away. I don't think they really would have been able to notice I had leprosy, but I felt like that—what if they know?"

Around that same time, however, he got to know a particular prostitute— another fellow Tamilian—who lived on the Mahim side of Dharavi, Bombay's biggest and most famous slum area.[5] "I was wandering around there on my own one day, and there were four or five prostitutes' houses there, and girls from each of them were calling out to me to come over. And this one girl, I didn't ever know her name, she was calling out in Tamil, and so we got in to conversation. I asked her where she came from, that kind of thing, and we discovered we were from the same part of Tamil Nadu."

Unlike in Grant Road, the prostitutes there didn't live in groups but in their own homes and, if there were pimps, they were not in evidence. The Tamil girl lived with her grandmother and other family members, "in a hut by the railway gates, with Mahim on one side, Dharavi on the other. If you went and visited her briefly, maybe it cost Rs20. But if you stayed the whole night, had sex once or twice and ate food there, it would cost around Rs100. I might have stayed over a few times, although I didn't take food there. Even in Bombay, I wouldn't like to take food unless I knew the people quite well. Maybe they were non-vegetarian households, we can't necessarily tell. But I'd drink coffee with them, or a cool drink. I probably only visited four or five times, usually if I was feeling sad or lonely. Just occasionally, when the police might have been torturing us or when there wasn't much going on, when I got to thinking, 'Oh! I'm so alone! Why do I have to sleep out here on my own on the pavements!,' those kinds of thoughts, then I'd go and visit her and I'd feel a bit better." It interested me, this story, not least because it

showed that while he clung on to the idea of avoiding cooked and inappropri-
ate foods from non-Brahmins, he did not consider sex with a non-Brahmin
polluting in the same way. Or perhaps it was that a continuation of his earlier
eating habits was more a matter of personal identity than of pollution and
purity. Certainly Das seemed to see it that way: "We weren't thinking much
of caste when I lived on the stations," he said, "and also I was a leprosy
patient, so why would I be concerned? I just look back and remember those
times, that's all. I don't make much of a judgement on them. In one way, I
feel very proud. I survived, and I lived and experienced all kinds of lives. In
another way though, I also feel very bad. I think, oh my God, I was born into
a Brahmin caste, to a good family, and then all these things happened to me!"
The story also interested me because it revealed more of a sadness than Das's
reminisces usually let on. He was free, it was true, but that rootlessness also
left him feeling alone and vulnerable.

Between sex and gambling, money came and went in easy fashion. There
was no point in sleeping out with wads of cash in your pocket because, as
Das explained it, the chances were you would be robbed or beaten for the
money by the station authorities or the police in any case. And arrest, as Das
learned, was always a possibility, lurking not very far in the background.
"We'd be sleeping there on the platform, and suddenly we'd be woken up by
the police vans—not the local railway police, other, more powerful ones—
and they would round some of us up and arrest us as suspects, although what
we were suspected of I was never sure. They'd get an order from the magis-
trates to keep us on remand, and we'd be put in jail for fifteen days while we
waited for the court hearings."

"We'd feel disorientated because we'd just been woken up, and they'd
throw us in the van, and fire questions and orders at us: 'Name? Do you have
any money on you? Sit there!' Things like that. And when we got to the
place, they'd check if we had any money hidden anywhere. We'd have to
remove our clothes and squat on the ground so they could check we weren't
stashing money in our buttocks. They would order us to squat and stand,
squat and stand . . . if anyone had anything hidden up there it would soon
work its way out! Then we'd be put into the cell."

The cell, as Das described it, was a single large room containing thirty or
forty prisoners, "with some kind of pot for passing motions in case we
needed to defecate during the night, but for urination we had to use the floor
at one end, where there would have been some holes in the wall for drainage.
Everyone tried to stay as close to the other end as possible!" Other facilities
were also minimal: 'We slept on the floor, which was fine, and from what I
can remember there weren't blankets or anything, and no fans. This was a
prison, not a lodge! There were certainly lots of mosquitoes."

The day-to-day routines were not so dissimilar to those Das had experienced earlier in the leprosy hospital, although sanitation there had been

slightly better. "In the mornings, the warders would come and shout at us to wake up, and we'd have to sing some Gandhian song—that was the morning prayer—and then we'd go out into the courtyard for breakfast." This was usually a form of *kanji*—the thick, starchy liquid produced from boiling rice or wheat—while other meals consisted of two chapattis and dhal-based curries. "We mainly got *sambar* and that kind of food—vegetables boiled up for a long time. It wasn't very good food, but it was edible, not too bad. The jailers also had to eat the same stuff so it couldn't be too awful. And special people—those who had money and could pay some bribes—they might have got some fried vegetable curries as well."

There was also work to do, but only for a few hours a day. "We'd be asked to do sweeping, pick weeds, whatever it might be. Then at 10am, when it was getting hot, we'd go back inside and have some rest." If other friends from the station had witnessed the raid they might have visited—Das was unsure whether his memories were intermingled with later incarcerations in Madras—but most of his company during those days in jail came from fellow porters who had been rounded up at the same time. His overwhelming emotion in describing his experience of prison, though, appears to be one of passive acceptance—embodied by a shrug of the shoulders—rather than, as I might have expected, a sense of fury at the injustice of what had happened. Even my horror at the unsanitary conditions he described was met with slightly amused puzzlement. What, he asked me incredulously, did I expect a prison to be like? "I wasn't much bothered," he said when I pressed him further on his response to those conditions. Even if they confirmed his expectations, surely his experiences there were at least unpleasant? But he refused to be drawn into my own reading of the situation: "I'd just sit there and think, okay, this is the way it is, this is the kind of life I have now. I made no fuss and, if the rowdies noticed me, I'd tell them I had leprosy, and they left me alone. The disease had its uses.[6] And the time passed and we were released, and things went on as before."

"After court they hadn't anything on us, so they couldn't keep us there. We went off to Bycula Station, near the jail, and just caught the train back to Dadar. I went to see my friends, got some money from them, took a bath, ate some tiffins and drank a tea, and started work again. What else could we do?"

Responding to his own question, he went on: "What was the use of being angry? What other choices did we have? If they'd beaten us badly, that would have been something else. But this was bearable. Sometimes they'd round you up and you'd escape, so those times you'd count yourself lucky. Sometimes you weren't so lucky, but those officers, if they catch you and put you in the cell, well, that's the job they have to do, their duty. It's not a personal thing against you. Other people, they might make a drama out of all this, but I'd just think of all the times I'd been lucky. Sometimes I'd been captured and told them I had leprosy, and they'd push me away and tell me to run off. That happened *so* many times. It was out of compassion mainly, I think, but there was also a bit of fear there. Some of them would feel: 'Ugh! You dirty fellow! I don't want to spoil my own life by having you close to me, so get away!'" And if Dadar became a difficult place to be, there was always the option of going to Bombay Central for a while, where Das knew Gopal and had made other friends.

In a way, the discovery that he had leprosy, a condition which, as it was widely understood at the time, debarred him from participation in marriage and other routine social expectations, was also liberating, and this was perhaps also part of the reason why Das remained so seemingly unmoved by his experience of prison. "There was no house, no family to worry about," he said nostalgically. "So when we went to sleep on the station we could automatically get to sleep easily, and wake up refreshed. Nowadays it's so much harder—so many dreams, so many worries to keep us awake at night! It was a very different kind of life we had on the station. On one side there was enjoyment and fun. Eating, playing cards, chatting, gambling, that kind of thing. On another side there's no worries, no wife and children to provide for, no parents around to obey. And on another side there were a few difficulties, the risk of being beaten or of being taken away by the police; and also some sadness, wondering what happened to your mother and father and your other family members. But if you're not bothering yourself too much with those things, if you're simply thinking, 'okay, my life is over, so I'll see what happens,' then, actually, it becomes all right. You can manage, you can survive fairly easily."

And so life went on for a few years, until, in 1974, Das decided to head back to Tamil Nadu. "I wanted a change," he said simply. "I thought, if I'm going to die, I will die there. It's my place." His thoughts about his own mortality were brought to the fore not by the fact he had leprosy, which appeared to have been having little physical effect that Das was aware of, but by a near miss on one of the trains. "I was jumping on a train to grab some seats for a passenger one time," he said, "and I missed, slipped down between the train and the platform, right up to my chin, and the train was still moving at quite a speed. Some how, I managed to pull myself up. I just had some scratches and bruises, and I still managed to get on and bag two seats! But it scared me, the pressure was increasing, and so I started thinking, okay, I'll go to Madras for a change. And if I have an accident there and am not so lucky, then at least I'll be in my home place."

"There were no big fights with other people, no big drama," he said. "I just told a few people I was going, bought a ticket—because I happened to have some money in my pocket at the time—and got myself a single seat on the train. It left in the afternoon, I arrived the next evening back in Madras, and got down and found a place to sleep the rest of the night. Then, the next day, I started out my life on Madras Central station again!"

NOTES

1. See, for an overview of discussions about gender roles in South Asia, Patricia Jeffery, *Frogs in a Well. Indian Women in Purdah* (London: Zed Press, 1979); Lynne Bennett, *Dangerous Wives and Sacred Sisters: Social and Symbolic Roles of High Caste Women in Nepal* (New York: Columbia University Press, 1983); Nivedita Menon, ed., *Gender and Politics in India* (Oxford: Oxford University Press, 1999); Cecilia Busby, *The Performance of Gender: An Anthropology of Everyday Life in a South Indian Fishing Village* (New Brunswick: Althone Press, 2000); Sarah Lamb, *White Saris and Sweet Mangoes: Aging, Gender, and Body in North India* (Berkeley: University of California Press, 2000); Linda Stone and Caroline James, "Dowry, Bride-Burning, and Female Power in India," *Women's Studies International Forum* 18, 2 (1995): 125–43. For more on changing gender roles in an increasingly globalizing India, see, for example, Smitha Radhakrishnan, *Appropriately Indian: Gender and Culture in a New Transnational Class* (Durham NC: Duke University Press, 2011) and Henrike Donner, *Domestic Goddesses: Maternity, Globalization and Middle-class Identity in Contemporary India* (Farnham: Ashgate, 2008).

2. To put Das's responses to his diagnosis of leprosy into comparative perspective, in addition to examples in Staples, *Peculiar People, Amazing Lives*, see Cassandra White, *An Uncertain Cure: Living with Leprosy in Rio de Janeiro* (New Brunswick, New Jersey: Rutgers University Press, 2009); Eric Silla, *People are Not the Same: Leprosy and Identity in Twentieth-Century Mali* (Oxford: James Currey, 1998); or—geographically closer—M. H. de Bruin, *Leprosy in South India: Stigma and Strategies of Coping* (Pondy Paper in Social Sciences: Institute Francais de Pondicherry, 1996).

3. For more on begging see James Staples, "Leprosy and Alms collecting in Mumbai," in *Livelihoods at the Margins,* ed. James Staples (Walnut Creek, California: Left Coast Press, 2007) 163–186; Ian McIntosh and Angus Erskine, " 'Money for nothing'? Understanding giving to beggars," *Sociological Research Online* 5, 1 (2000), http://www.socresonline.org.uk/5/1/mcintosh.html; L. Navon, "Beggars, metaphors and stigma," *Social History of Medicine,* 11(1998): 89–105.

4. Cross-checks with internet and newspaper sources appear to confirm the details of Das's account of Matka. See, for example, Shailendra Awasthi, "From Matka king to anonymous punter, life's come a full circle for him," *Express India* (December 2, 2007), accessed May 29, 2013, http://expressindia.indianexpress.com/latest-news/From-Matka-king-to-anonymous-punter-lifes-come-a-full-circle-for-him/245717/

5. For background on Dharavi, see Kalpana Sharma, *Rediscovering Dharavi: Stories from Asia's Largest Slum* (New Delhi: Penguin India, 2000).

6. See, for examples of the uses leprosy might be put to by those afflicted with the condition, James Staples, "Disguise, Revelation and Copyright: Disassembling the South Indian Leper," *Journal of the Royal Anthropological Institute* (N.S.), 9 (2003): 295–315; James Staples, Delineating disease: self-management of leprosy identities in South India," *Medical Anthropology* 23, 1 (2004): 69–88. For an account of the positive uses of negative identities more generally—and the conundrums thus presented—see Jonathan Parry, "The Koli Dilemma," *Contributions to Indian Sociology* (N.S.) 4 (1970): 84–104.

Chapter Four

Reunions

It was good to be back on familiar soil and to fill his lungs with Tamil air. Das had been away for six years, but not that much had changed on the station. Several people he had known from his time there in 1968 were still there doing the same kind of things, including Kamala, who still sat behind her makeshift banana stall to one side of the main entrance. "We greeted each other and we talked sometimes," said Das, "but I'd been just a boy when I'd helped on her stall back then, and I was too old for that now. Anyway, her own son was growing up and he was out there working with her most of the time."

He got to know many people quite well on the station over the next few years, some of whom I met when I was subsequently with Das in Madras over the years and we needed help getting seats on trains. A few of them, or their descendants, were still there when we visited the station in July 2009 so that Das could walk me through, as well as talk to me about, the places where he spent his days.[1] There were a select few people, however, who he describes as "thick friends": those on whom he relied for support.

Manoj, a fellow unofficial porter, was one of his first friends on the station. Das was introduced to him by Kamala, whose banana stall was close to the pitch where Manoj's wife and her sister sold strings of jasmine, and it was his early support that protected Das against some of the other porters who may not have taken kindly to a new man muscling in on their territory. Manoj had been there a long time: station dwellers listened to what he had to say. Another friend, Mohammed from Kerala was also a porter. He was an unauthorized one, like Manoj, when Das first knew him, but later on he got "the badge" and donned the distinctive red uniform. "I was friendly with him from the early days," said Das, "and continued to see him on the platform now and then until he died in 2002. He was one of the head porters by the end. Once, when I was working in Anandapuram and we had some urgent parcels to send to Delhi, I went to ask him for advice on how best to get them there quickly. He told me not to worry about it, and without saying any more arranged it personally with one of the ticket collectors to get it on a train and delivered at the other end. He didn't take a single paise. This was more than ten years after I'd left the station, but we don't forget those who have looked out for us and have lived through the same types of problems. Like Manoj, Mohammed played cards and ate food with us—I suppose we were like a kind of family."[2]

"They were all normal, ordinary people, all there for different reasons," Das recalled, when I pressed him for more details on his friends' backgrounds. "A few of them lived outside and came to work in the station, but there was a core group of maybe ten or fifteen of us who lived by the station on the platform. They weren't educated, most of them, but they knew how to get by."

Life followed a routine similar to the one he had been used to on Dadar Station, although for Das, it was the food that most distinguished the two locations. "The culture's a bit different in Madras compared to Bombay," he said. "In Bombay we'd eat bread and things like that for breakfast, there were no real *tiffins* like there are in Madras: there, on the station, we could get good dosas, idlis and vadas, and proper sambar and chutneys too. It was also a lot cheaper in Madras: you could get the same amount of food for a fifth of the price it would have been in Bombay, so there was more money left over to spend on other things. Not that there was anything for me to save for, so I just spent more money on gambling, or on going to the cinema, that kind of thing. Drinking wasn't a habit I had at that time. I'd also buy lots of the cheap detective novels you can buy on the stands in the station, and read them in the afternoons, lying on bunks in trains before they were ready for going out. Like I said before, there's a risk if you keep too much money with you, so it was better to earn and spend, earn and spend. I lived for the moment. I used to think, even if I die now, at least it will be in my own place, Tamil Nadu. My friends here will take my body away somewhere and sort things out."

Betting on horse races, he learned on the station, was one of the most entertaining ways of spending money in Madras, although Das claimed he more often made a profit than a loss. "In Bombay," he said, "we had the *Matka,* or the numbers to pass the time. Here, I discovered the race track." It was a fellow Brahmin porter, known always simply as Mr Iyer, who first took him. After that it became a regular Saturday or Sunday activity. "We'd go in and get the book about the horses so we could study their form," he said. "I could read, which is why Iyer and some of my other friends liked having me along, even if I didn't have money to bet with. I'd read up on the horses' track records, on how many minutes and seconds they had taken to finish each of their previous races, what kind of distances they ran best over, any changes in their weights, who the jockey was. There were all sorts of calculations we could make."[3]

As a novice to horse racing when Das first took me, I was baffled by the acronyms and numbers that filled the pocket-sized race book we bought at the entrance. But Das, as it became very clear, was in his element. His eyes flitted quickly and expertly over the columns of tiny letters and numbers as he made calculations in his head and, within minutes, he declared the likely winners. He did not get it right every time, but more often than not his predicted winner would be in the top three. I was impressed. The problems, though, came when there was what Das called "an upset": when a favourite fell early on, or an unexpected contender took the lead.

There was other information, not included in the book, that was also useful to know, and Das kept up with it by following the racing news in the papers and on the radio. "Lots of the horses were owned by the major business men, and they'd set things up so they knew who was going to win. They might give Rs30 lakhs in gift money to an opponent to lose, for example— there was big money involved, so it was worth this investment—or maybe a pair of them would arrange it so the first man's horse won one race, the other one would win the next. Not cheating, exactly: they might just tell one of their jockeys not to try very hard. We reckoned they understood very well which races they would win, so we needed to look out for the patterns. Mr Iyer taught me all of those things, and although it was complicated I gradually understood how it worked. I got a reputation there for knowing who was likely to win! I'd have all sorts of people coming up and asking me: 'Subbaiah! Subbaiah! What's your choice? Who are you tipping to win this or that race?' I never told them my name or age or anything, so they just called me Subbaiah, and it became one of my names."

"One time my friend bet Rs240 for the jackpot—which means you need a winner in each race—and he won Rs120,000! All from one bet! He had to pay Rs48,000 tax, but he still got Rs72,000 in his pocket. He gave me Rs2,000 for helping him." Mostly the spoils were lower, but making money was not really an issue for Das in those days: "I'd go with just Rs100 in my pocket, whatever I had on me. I can't say I made a big profit, but maybe I broke even. And you'd get to spend the day there, have some food and so on, so it was worth it."

It was an easy way to pass time, as I found out for myself when Das took me to several race meetings in 2011, in Bangalore and Mumbai as well as Chennai. As soon as we were through the rusty turnstiles we were enveloped within a warm surge of humanity—or, at least, that part of it represented by Indian men. Women, even now, are relatively rare at the racecourse, especially outside Bombay. The colour usually provided in Indian crowd scenes by women in their bright saris and salwar kameez was noticeably absent: the greyness of the vista only occasionally broken by the incongruous presence of a saffron clad sadhu.

"Odd place for a renouncer to hang out," I commented.

"There are always a few here," said Das. "Maybe it helps when they don't care if they win or lose."

"Or maybe," he added, watching one of them draw deeply on his cheroot as he studied his race book, "they are just charlatans."

The air in the central hall—where the bookies operated from raised wooden cages, their odds chalked up on boards outside—was thick with tobacco smoke and the fragrance of betel nut. The floor, by the time we left, was also dense with spent betting slips, cigarette butts and the debris of a thousand *tiffins*. "But what's amazing about it," as Das pointed out, "is that you'll see everyone here, from rickshaw *wallahs* and station porters to Marwari business men and professionals. There's a private members" grandstand and places where not everyone can go, but mostly we're all together, doing the same thing. It doesn't matter who you are or where you come from." Even I did not get stared at. Nor, Das implied, would a vagrant leprosy patient. I was beginning to see the attraction, and that was even before the thrill of the race itself.

Back at the station, the few material things Das and his fellow station-dwellers possessed—clothes, mats and bedding and, in some cases, cooking vessels and plates—were kept in old trunk boxes up on the wall by the cycle rickshaw stand, sheltered by gnarled old peepal trees. The *maistry*, a Christian from Kerala called Maximillian, used to keep guard over them when they were away working. Das did not cook for himself—it was a skill he had always managed to avoid acquiring. But Manoj's wife cooked for her whole family, including her sister and their respective children, and Das would eat with them as long as the dishes were vegetarian. "They were quite rough, those platform people," he told me. "They were from very low castes—the equivalent of Madigas and Malas, most of them—and so bad language used to come very easily from their tongues! Brahmins don't know how to speak in that kind of way. But they were also good, kind people, and they always looked out for me." The food they prepared, unlike that which he would have eaten in his mother's house, was straightforward, too. It was cooked over open fires or on kerosene stoves not far from the station's borders in just two cooking pots—one for the rice and the other for the curry, usually lentils mixed with what ever vegetables were for sale on stalls close by, seasoned simply with salt, turmeric and chilli powder.

In the same way that neither caste nor religion seemed a particular bar to friendship among the pavement dwellers, leprosy did not appear to be an issue either. Like other diseases, it was perhaps more common among their group than among the general population. Manoj himself was a tuberculosis patient, and his family had also befriended and looked out for another leprosy affected boy, Raj, whose unwashed, dreadlocked hair, and face, disfigured by a raised skin rash and swelling around his eyes, disguised the fact that he was only eighteen or nineteen years old. He arrived on the station in the late 1970s, along with another, much older leprosy affected man, whose loss of fingers and toes and collapsed nose identified him much more obviously as a sufferer of the disease. Although they were avoided by others in mainstream society, those who lived on the station had little fear of contagion, whether spiritual or physical, and, as long as they did not cause them any problems, were content to accept them. Manoj and the others were, after all, already a group living on the peripheries of mainstream society. For Das's own part, he anyway had few outward signs that he had ever had leprosy. His legs and feet were dry and the skin on them cracked, and his toe and finger nails thicker and darker than they otherwise would have been, but to the untrained eye they would not have betrayed his status. He had, he said, been lucky. He had also taken another course of treatment from the nearby hospital after his arrival on the station and, when they tested him, the reading showed him to be clear. He was unsure if he believed it—nor, really, what it meant, since he had not by then accepted that leprosy was curable—but he must have been conscious that his body continued to function as it always had done.

In terms of his routine, Das did much the same as he had done on Dadar station. "On an average kind of day, I'd wake up at around 5am for the Howrah Mail, then the Circa Express, then the Hyderabad Express, the Grand Trunk Express . . . and so on, like that. There were plenty of trains to choose from. And if I could get passengers on two or three of them I'd be happy. In particular, I was interested in getting the passengers who were looking for hotels, because they brought in the most money and the work was easier too. I didn't like having to carry heavy loads of luggage if I could avoid it. I could speak some English, and some Hindi and Marathi now, as well, so I'd especially seek out travellers from other states and foreigners to work with. I wanted to improve myself, and I thought there was more dignity in being a guide for people—taking them to hotels or to see the sights—than there was in carrying their bags and suitcases around, so that was my aim. And because I'd lived in other places and had these languages, I had an advantage over some of the porters."

"One time," he remembered, "this man from Singapore arrived on the station. He was from Tamil Nadu originally, but he hadn't been back for a long time, I don't think. He was there with his wife and their small child, they'd come directly from the airport, and they wanted to get the train to Hyderabad, overnight. I saw them standing there looking out of place on the platform, so I went and asked them if I could help and he told me his problem: he didn't care how much he had to pay, but he needed to get to Hyderabad. They had tickets already, he said, but no berth reservations, and they'd just flown in so they were tired and needed to rest. So I said, okay, come with me and we'll find the ticket collector (TC), which we did. But the TC told us there was nothing else that night with space on it going to Hydera-bad, so I started trying to convince the passenger that it would be better to go the next day. 'You look tired,' I said, 'Let me take you to a nice hotel and you and the family can get some rest. Then we'll work on getting you a reservation for tomorrow. It will be easy enough: you're non-resident so if need be we can try for the foreigners' quota.' I convinced him this was the best idea and took him and his wife and child to a hotel, and said I'd be back in the morning to get their tickets sorted out, and that I'd stay with them if they wanted and see them on to the train. They booked an expensive room, and gave me Rs100 for taking them and their bags there, and the hotel gave me another Rs150 in commission. I went back to the station and cashed in the old tickets they'd given me, which weren't useful to them any more. I managed to get Rs200 back on them—so that was Rs450 already. Not bad, no?"

"Then, in the morning, I called in at the hotel for them, had some breakfast with them and we chatted. He asked me where I was from and what my education was, and I explained that I was educated to tenth standard and had then run away after a fight with my family. That was my standard explanation if people asked me. Then we went to the reservations counter at the station and I sorted them out berths in the air conditioned carriage, took them back to the hotel again, and then picked them up when it was time for them to go. And when I put him on the train, he got out his wallet and gave me Rs700! I couldn't believe it! I'd made over Rs1,000 for just that small amount of work, and they'd given me breakfast in their hotel, too! At other times, you'd have to fight and haggle to get just Rs10 out of a passenger, but you'd get good ones like this man from Singapore in between, and then times were good!"

Das was on familiar territory now, so he also felt able to branch out to offer sightseeing trips around the city as an additional service. "I'd meet people off the train from North India who weren't familiar with the south, so I'd try to convince them to stay in one of the hotels that paid good commission and, when I was taking them there, would have the chance to tell them about all the places I could take them to see in Madras, if they wanted: Mount Road, for shopping or to drink lime sodas in Spencer's, the old department store before it burned down, or to the beach, perhaps? I knew these places already so it was no trouble to take them there, and useful for them too."

"Some people would be on the way to Mahabalipuram to see the shore temples and the rock carvings—it's only an hour or so further down the coast on the bus—and if that was the case I'd take them to the bus stand and get them on to the bus. You have to push and shove to get on and get a seat sometimes, but I was good at doing that. A couple of times, I also accompanied tourists there as a guide: the first group were North Indians, Hindi speakers; the second was a white couple, from England or Germany or somewhere, and they spoke English." Das had never been to Mahabalipuram before he took tourists there, but he knew some of the history from school, and had become adept at glossing over gaps in his knowledge. "I knew that it had been developed as a port hundreds of years ago by the Pallavas, and that they had left behind caves and temples and wall carvings, telling Mahabharata stories. But that was enough. There were signs in Tamil next to everything, so I read them quickly to myself and then translated the information to the tourists, so they thought I knew what I was talking about. Then we'd go and have a look at the beach, at the sea, and finally have something to eat at a restaurant before heading back. It was like being a tourist without any of the costs!"

For an experienced porter, passengers were easy to predict: "We'd just need to study them for a few moments," said Das, "and we'd be able to tell from the look of them and the way they behaved whether they had much knowledge of Madras or not. North Indians you could tell by the paleness of their skin and their clothing, and foreigners you could always spot. Once we knew they needed help, we just had to convince them we were the people to give it. And once we'd got them on our side, they wouldn't want to leave us. They'd rely on us to help them, sort everything out. So life was mostly quite enjoyable, and there was enough money floating around to get by. If I didn't feel like working for a day or two—if I was sick or something—that was okay too: I knew the *chai wallahs* and the man who ran the *tiffin*s stall, so they'd give me credit. There were no worries there."

Das also had experience of foreigners from Bombay to draw upon. Their numbers were not vast, but the hippy trails of the 1960s and 1970s washed up a fair share of overseas travellers through India's major cities, and Das and his friends were well placed to make the most of them. "All I knew about them was that they had money to spend. We used to say, in Tamil, whether they come from Britain, Australia or Japan we couldn't tell: they are all white people, but they all have money, so why should we care? I can't mirror their pronunciation, but if they spoke English I could make out what they said and I could answer them."

Das, who was telling me this part of the story over thirty years later as we sipped hot sweet tea on the verandah of the village house where I was staying, started laughing to himself at this point. He paused for a moment and looked a little sheepish. "It's . . ." he paused again. "I'm not sure if I should say the next bit!" I was intrigued, but sat quietly and waited to see what he would say next. "Okay, I will tell you!" he decided finally, and took a deep breath before continuing with his story. "One day, when I was in Madras Central station, I met this white foreigner. He was about thirty, I think, older than I was at the time, probably younger than you are now. And you must remember, I didn't look like I do now. I was good looking and everything: fair-skinned, slim, and I kept my hair and my moustache well combed and all. And this foreigner, he told me he'd already booked a room at the Woodlands hotel, and he asked me to come back there with him. Lots of foreigners used to stay there. I didn't know why he wanted me to go there, but I thought, why not? So we got there, and he asked me if I wanted to do anything: eat some food maybe."

"I said yes, that would be good, and he ordered some paper *dosa*s, cooked with ghee. Only in Madras can you get such good paper *dosas*—wider than the table, usually! While we were waiting for them to come, he suggested to me that I could go and have a bath. I thought that was a funny thing to ask me to do, but then I thought, why not? It's a good opportunity to have a bath in a better place than usual. And there was a bucket of hot water, good foreign soap and a thick towel, so I spent a while in there! When I came out the food had arrived, so I sat down on the bed with the towel around me and enjoyed the paper *dosa*. There was sambar, good potato curry, and three chutneys: mint, coconut and chilli; green, white and orange, like the Indian flag. And then . . . how can I say?" Das paused to laugh sheepishly again and he looked down at his floor, avoiding eye contact with me. He was more comfortable talking about the chutneys than other aspects of the encounter. "I mean, nothing happened, but he was looking at me, and I understood then that maybe he wanted something more than to eat with me. He wanted to touch me, I think. Maybe I guessed it earlier but tried not to think about it. I wasn't interested to have sex with a man. Anyway, I thought to myself, I'll just finish my food and then I'll think of a reason why I have to go. But then he came and sat a bit closer to me, and he was looking at me very intensely, so I moved away a bit and said, 'Actually, suddenly I'm not feeling at all well, I think I've got some fever and dizziness, so I don't think I should do anything else today. I'm sorry. We'll see later, another time, maybe?' And he was very kind to me. He looked concerned and he said, 'Oh dear, you sit there and have some rest. Can I get you some medicine?' I said no, but he gave me some money to get some medication anyway—Rs200, I think it was—and as I went he told me that he'd be there for three months, so I could go to visit him anytime. 'Okay,' I said, 'I'll come back when I'm feeling better.' But I never did! I went to the bathroom to finish getting dressed, and then I left as quickly as I could!"

Other encounters were more to Das's liking, even though he spoke of them as if they were entirely beyond his control. As he had already made clear, things happened to him rather than as a consequence of his own actions. Having got out of the way the awkward story of how he had found himself wearing nothing more than a towel on the hotel bed of a foreign man with designs on him, he was keen to download more details of sexual escapades. There was doubtless something cathartic about telling these long hidden stories. But, as Das expressed it, they were also an essential part of what life on the station was like, and, without them, he felt his story would lack authenticity. "Why do I tell you these things?" he asked, partly rhetorically, but partly because he was trying to figure out the answer for himself. "You know, these things are not easily shared with other people. I haven't really told them to anyone else before. But this is what life on the platform is like, what it's really like. Somebody might say differently, and different people will have different experiences, but this is my experience, it is my history, my story, so I want to tell it to you fully and truthfully. You can put in polite words and other things for me, but I want to say what really happened to me."

The other incident he told me about that afternoon had taken place at the nurses' home near the station, again in the mid-1970s. There was a big government hospital directly opposite Madras Central Station—it is still there today—and the staff accommodation was close by. "They'd come in from the villages, those nurses, most of them young and unmarried, and they'd all live here together in those quarters. We'd often take them and their luggage there when they got down from the train. They'd ask me to take their trunk or suitcase, and put it in their room. Now remember, at that time I was still looking good—I wasn't dark skinned like I am now, from the sun and the leprosy drugs. And I didn't look like the other leprosy patients on the station. I was a good-looking boy, around twenty-four years old or so."

"And one day I took this nurse back to her quarters, to this room she shared with three or four other nurses, but they were all out on duty in the hospital at that time, so when we got there it was just me and her. She said to the watchman, on the way up, 'He'll just bring my luggage for me, and then I'll send him back down, okay?' But when we got there, she immediately locked the door behind us. 'What are you doing?' I asked her, but she just put her finger to her lips and cautioned me to be quiet. 'You sit there,' she commanded, so I did, 'and I'll get the money to pay you.' And then she turned around and opened her dress, so I could see her breasts and everything, and she started coming towards me. She was older than me, about thirty. She was plump and dark skinned, probably low caste I think; lots of converted Christians from those castes became nurses. 'If you're not making love to me,' she said, 'I will shout and scream and say that you tried to rape me.' Just like that! So what can I do? We didn't have to worry about AIDS and other things back in those days, and I was young, so it wasn't a problem. I had sex with her and, afterwards, she paid me Rs100 for carrying her luggage there, and she showed me the way downstairs again.

"The watchman came out and said, 'What happened up there? Why did you take so long dropping off a piece of luggage?' And she said to him not to worry, that something in her room was broken, and that she'd asked me to fix it for her while I was there. He said: 'But why? There's an odd jobs man here who could have done that repair for you.' I quickly replied back: 'No, no, but she needed it done very urgently sir!' And as I spoke she leant across and gave him Rs20. He just took the money, raised his eyebrows a bit and turned away as he stuffed the note into his pocket. 'Okay then, go,' he said to me, and I was off. After I told the other porters on the station about what had happened they were all very keen to carry the nurses' luggage back to the nurses' home for them, but it didn't ever happen again, at least not for me."

Fun though Das made life sound in those pre-AIDS days, those who lived on the station also faced the same harsh realities that he had faced back in Bombay. "Sometimes, touting for business, people would speak rudely to us or shout. We were open targets, living out there by the station. And sometimes there were also fights and other things, especially with the authorities, but sometimes with passengers too. In fact, sometimes we'd try to make arguments with the passengers just so that we can push them to give us more money. That side of things was always more ugly. Sometimes, in the festival seasons, when the trains were all too full, they'd pay us just to get them on the train at all, not even a seat. So we'd open the door and ram them in first, and then we'd pass in the suitcase. Once the passenger was on, having already agreed a price of Rs100, we might say, okay, give me Rs200! We didn't do that much, just occasionally. And they'd get angry and say, 'But you told me Rs100!' What can they do about it though? They are on the train and can't get off without losing their space. And we're on the platform with their luggage in hand!"

Then, one afternoon in 1976, Das was sleeping in the general compartment of a train in a siding that had not yet been put back out for service. "I was asleep, and it all happened very quickly," he said, "I'd been reading a Tamil detective novel and had dozed off, and when I was awoken I just reacted to protect myself. This policeman was walking up and down the train, clearing people out, and he saw me sleeping on one of the bunks. So he came at me with this thick wire flex that he'd got from somewhere, and lashed it down on me. It felt worse than being hit by one of their *lathis* [sticks]. I woke up from the stinging pain across my face and chest, and saw him standing there over me, his face all contorted and his arm raised back, still holding up the flex, ready to strike for a second time, and I leapt back in shock. I was shaking with pain and anger. I leapt down from the train and just there in front of me was a big iron rod, so, without thinking, I grabbed it up, clambered back on to the train, where he was still walking down the central aisle, looking for more of us to beat, and I rushed up behind him and brought the rod down hard on the back of his head. I didn't think about it, I just did it. There was a horrible cracking sound, he fell to the ground and there was blood pumping out everywhere! I was terrified. What had I done? So I dropped the rod and turned and ran away as fast as I could, and absconded for a couple of weeks."

"I was almost too scared to come back," Das went on, "but when I did I discovered that at least he had survived: he just had to get some stitches in his head, so I didn't have a murder charge on me! And one of my friends, while I was away, had made a compromise with him. 'Why did you beat him?' he had asked the policeman, 'He's a leprosy patient, a Brahmin boy, an educated boy, and you should have left him alone. If it was money you were after you should have just come and asked him for it. One of us will give it to you.' And they paid him off, I think."

Das had got away lightly, particularly given that the incident had happened at the height of the state of Emergency, which ran from June 1975 to March 1977. The Emergency features only in passing in Das's account of his life, even though some of the events he described might well have been a direct result of it. Nationally, events had come to a head in early June 1975, when the Prime Minister, Indira Gandhi, was found guilty by the courts of misusing Government resources in her election campaign. Although she had been cleared of much more serious charges, the ruling nevertheless ejected her from her parliamentary seat and banned her from running for office for six years. It was in order to avoid this that, two weeks later on June 25, India's President, Fakhuruddin Ali Ahmed, declared, at his prime minister's behest, a state of emergency. The reasons she cited for it—and continued to cite as it was extended at regular interviews until a general election finally took place nearly two years later in March 1977—were threats to national security from Pakistan, and anti-Government strikes and protests which threatened the stability of India. [4]

Protest leaders up and down the country were rounded up and thrown into jail without trial. Civil liberties were suspended, and the prime minister ruled not through parliament but through decree. In Tamil Nadu, one of the few states where Gandhi's party, the Congress, had not been in charge at the time, the authority of the elected chief minister was side-stepped through the imposition of President's rule. Specifically, this meant the dismissal of M Karnnanidhi, leader of the Dravida Munnetra Kazhagaru (DMK), a party calling for local rather than Delhi-centred power.

Das, however, appeared only partially aware of the extraordinary political events that were unfolding around him, despite the fact that he was one of the estimated 140,000 people who were arrested and imprisoned without trial during that period. "We'd often go to the local cinema in Tambaram, thirty-odd kilometres out of town on the train," Das recalled. "It was cheaper there than the city cinemas, just a thatch roofed place with an earth floor and simple benches to sit on. You could watch two films for thirty paise, and the last one didn't finish until around 3am, so it was also a good place to get some sleep without being disturbed. Some of us would go there once or twice a week in the early days, then wait on the benches at the station for the first train back to the city."

"But one time we were waiting there at Tambaram station—it would have been about 3:30am—when a van load of policemen suddenly appeared, and started rounding us up. I think they had quotas of arrests to make and must have been falling behind that month, so we were all arrested under the Indian penal code on suspicion of wrong-doing. They never told us what we were suspected of. We were just put in prison on remand for a couple of weeks."

After his experience in Bombay, however, being locked away for a while without being told why seemed little more than an occupational hazard to Das. "These things happened whether there was the Emergency or not," he told me with a shrug. "Just like in Bombay, they rounded up some of us and took us away to the prison because we were under suspicion of having done something. But nothing came of it and we were released eventually. One thing I'd say, though, is that Bombay prisons are better. They were not as rough as the prisons in Madras. There, you saw the older, longer term and more experienced prisoners cheating and mistreating the newer ones, bullying them. But no-one bothered me much in either place. In both prisons I just sat it out and thought, okay, this is one kind of life, so be it. We were just small people, what could we do to change things?"

"Looking back, there were probably more police around at that time, and they were more troublesome than they had been in the past, which is why the incident with the iron rod happened. But I never thought much about why that should be so. We weren't interested in politics, and we didn't think about it like that, either. We'd just think, perhaps, why are the police doing this or that? But usually we didn't bother. We just thought about what we needed to do to manage the situation, whatever it was."

The emergency period was also the time when, famously, the euphemistically titled family planning program, under the control of the prime minister's son, Sanjay Gandhi, became a front for thousands of forced vasectomies.[5] Many of those I worked with over the years told me tales of farm laborers being collected from the fields by local officials and taken off in vans or on the backs of ox-carts to makeshift family planning centres where, whether they wanted them or not, and whether they had any children already or not, they were operated upon. Some of the older men I spoke to were only spared because they told the officials they had leprosy, and so did not plan to have children in any case. The strategy probably only worked because the officials were afraid of contracting the disease themselves.

Das's vasectomy, too, occurred during the emergency period, but—as a single man whose aspirations to have children had already been curtailed—it was not an event that overly traumatized him. "I was outside the station somewhere, drinking tea at a tea stall on my own," he recalled, "when a man came up and started talking to me. He was friendly enough, but he also asked lots of questions: who was I? Was I married or unmarried? Where did I live? He said he worked for the government, and that I needed to go for a medical check-up of some kind, but that it was nothing to worry about, and that he would take me there for it himself. I was a bit suspicious, but he kept pressing me, and he said that I'd even get some money for it, as an incentive.

"I think I only worked out what was happening when we got to the hospital and I was talking to some of the other men in the waiting room. But I didn't make a fuss. I didn't think I could have children anyway, being a leprosy patient, so I thought it was probably better to have the operation and be done with it. The agent, the man who took me there, he was paid something, and I got something too, so I suppose everyone was happy with the outcome!"

Much more important to Das than seemingly abstract decisions taken thousands of miles away in Delhi—even when he bore the brunt of some of those decisions—were more personally life-changing events, one of which occurred toward the end of 1979. It was, indeed, one of the three pivotal events—the first being the discovery he had leprosy, the third yet to come—that recur in even the most synoptic accounts of Das's life.

Manoj's wife and her sister had been sitting, cross-legged on their mat, stringing together flowers to make garlands for sale, in the shade of two peepal trees—so big and old that their roots were pulling up the pavement beneath them—on the corner of the cycle rickshaw stand outside the station. They were chatting to Raj, the other leprosy patient, when Das got there, bemoaning the fact that he lived under the shadow of the older man. "He wasn't very clean or well-kept, that old patient," Das said, "and he was a bit of a rowdy, drinking fellow. Rough, even by the standards of Manoj's family! This younger boy, although he was unkempt too, was very timid, and I don't think they liked him being under that fellow's control. They wanted to hear him speak for himself." Das joined them, and their idle chatter gave way to a few rounds of the car number game—which, like all the games Das played—involved gambling. "We'd pick a number, and the first person to get five passing cars with that number as the last number on the plate would win the pot. We'd put on Rs50 for five cars, say, or Rs100 for ten. It was a simple game, just there to pass the time."

"As we played it," Das went on, "I started to chat to this Raj fellow. He told me his name was actually Chandra Prakash, that he, like me, was a Brahmin, and that his native place was Kumbakonam. 'Oh,' I said, 'my family lived there for sometime, after they shifted from the village'—which I gave the name of—and he said, 'Oh yes? I've heard of that village, my mother also came from there.' That's a coincidence, I thought, so I asked him what his father's name was. 'Gajavakra,' he said. 'That's my father's name too!' I replied, but it was a fairly common name in Tamil Nadu, so I asked him what his mother's name was, and when he said 'Subbalakshmi,' I knew for sure. There couldn't have been two couples in that village called Gajavakra and Subbalakshmi, who had two sons called Mohandas and Chandra

Prakash. 'Then you're my brother!' I shouted out, and we embraced each other, right there under the two trees. Both of us were weeping. The women who were there couldn't believe it either: they dropped the flowers they were threading together and wept with joy for us. It was like a scene from a cinema movie! We hadn't seen each other for ten years or so, and Chandra Prakash had been such a small boy when I left. Leprosy had changed his face, too, and the way he wore his hair, unbrushed and unwashed, made him look different. I'd known there was something familiar about him, but I would never have guessed he was my brother!"

Manoj's wife and sister-in-law were insistent, now that Chandra Prakash had been identified as Das's brother, that he should be taken under their wing and away from the guardianship of the older leprosy patient. "They called him there, that patient, and told him what we had discovered, said that they would be caring for him from now on. Then we got him bathed, had his hair washed and cut, and got him into some clean clothes. You could still tell he had leprosy, but he looked much better. I think that before then, he was too afraid to get close to other people: he knew he had leprosy, and, like me, he thought that was the end, and that he'd better stay only around patients, which is why he'd stuck with that fellow. He'd arrived at the station after wandering here and there, and also like me he'd gone inside to carry luggage, but he wasn't much good at getting the seats and other things. I'd sent him once to grab a seat—this was before we knew we were brothers—but he was too timid to fight for a place, he wouldn't have been able to make a living doing that!"

Their stories of what had happened to them since their separation at the end of 1968 unfolded over the next few days, although I also had some separate interviews with Chandra Prakash to get his side of the story. He had gone, when his father absconded, to live with the oldest of his paternal uncles, the Tamil Pandit, in Trichy. It was another two or three months before word got back to his mother, by then in Bombay with Parvathi and her family, that Gajavakra had absconded, and by that time Chandra Prakash was settled and studying in a local school. With Gajavakra gone and Chandra Prakash taken care of, she stayed on in Bombay to help Parvathi take care of her children. Over the course of the next year, however, Gajavakra's brother developed problems of his own: his wife fell sick, and it was becoming difficult to care for his own children, let alone his brother's son. "He wrote then to my mother in Bombay," Chandra Prakash remembers, "telling her to come to Trichy to help. She wrote back saying that she couldn't leave Bombay at that time because Parvathi wasn't well enough and she had too much work to do there. So he wrote again and told her, okay, if you can't come and help us, why should we take care of your son? You can take him back!"

Subbalakshmi agreed, and Chandra Prakash's uncle dispatched him on a train back to Madras, from where another relative, Parvathi's brother's daughter, collected him and accompanied him on another train to the family home. Chandra Prakash stayed there for around year with his mother, at their large rented house in thirteenth road, Chembur, where he attended fourth class. He found school difficult, mainly because of the language differences: he'd never studied Hindi and he had no Marathi to fall back on. The family also decided that he was getting rather old still to be in fourth class. He was over ten years old already. An alternative route would be for him to learn the mantras, part of the thinking in leaving him with his uncle in the first place, so that he could help officiate with the priest at Hindu life cycle rituals. As the pandit in his own family was no longer in a position to help him, they needed to find an alternative route.

Subrahmanyam, by luck, knew a priest from Kanchipuram—one of Tamil Nadu's foremost temple cities—who had been in Bombay conducting pujas for several Tamil families, their own included. The priest agreed to take Chandra Prakash back with him, and to enrol him in the "mantras school"—as Chandra Prakash referred to it—with which he was involved. "He lived at the school too, and went off to visit people on special occasions and festivals to do pujas for them," he explained. "I stayed in the hostel for the boys who were also training to do that work. It was a good time, a happy life." He spent a year there, then shifted to another, new school that they had opened in Bangalore. When the Bangalore school failed to get enough entrants and had to close down, he was shifted again to another branch in Salem, back in central Tamil Nadu. He never returned to Bombay in all that three-year period—it was seen as a long way in those days—but Subrahmanyam did send him spending money and clothes every now and then."

When he was studying at Salem, one of the teachers noticed a patch on his back, and sent him to have it tested at the doctors. It was leprosy. There was no dramatic banishment from the school—Chandra Prakash was told he could return if he got treatment and his patches cleared up—but it was made clear he could not continue with his training. "I told them I didn't know where my father was and that my mother was far away in Bombay, so they wrote to one of my father's other brothers—the second one, my small father—who was living and working in Kumbakonam. He came to collect me." This uncle was, as Chandra Prakash was well aware, one of the poorest members of the family: he made just Rs90 a month working in a meals hotel, and had a wife and four children of his own to support. But there was a leprosy hospital nearby, where they enrolled Chandra Prakash for treatment, and he began a course of Dapsone.

Aware of his uncle's financial position, he also realized he needed to find a way to contribute to the household income, and managed to find work helping a priest. "I helped him with weddings and other functions, because I knew well all the right pujas for each occasion, and by doing that I was able to pay my own way, to support myself within my uncle's family." This worked all right for a year or so, but then the priest died unexpectedly, and Chandra Prakash's source of additional income for the family was cut off. "I hadn't finished my treatment, I was supposed to keep going back to get the drugs and take them," he told me, "but I felt all right by then, so I didn't understand why I should: I thought it was probably okay to stop them. And I knew I needed to find a way of supporting myself, that it wasn't possible to stay at my uncle's house when he had so many already to feed and very little money, so I left without telling anyone and got the train to Trichy, where I found work in a meals hotel. No-one came after me: I'm sure they were relieved that the extra burden on them was lifted! I wasn't paid very well— just Rs22 a month—but I was a server and I got meals and *tiffins* there as well. It was okay, I liked it there, life was happy. But after three years, and having stopped taking my treatment, my disease was starting to come out again."

This time Chandra Prakash knew what it was, and so did his employers. Again, there was no dramatic end to his appointment: his boss just told him, quite gently, according to Chandra Prakash, that he would not be able to work there in that condition. He paid him off his salary and gave him a bit more. "They said that once I'd been treated, I could come back, but it wasn't good for me to be working there with this disease, that customers wouldn't like it," Chandra Prakash recalled. "But I didn't go back to the hospital then, I kept on working at different places—a few weeks in one place, a few weeks in another. But if I stayed any longer they always started to notice the signs that I had leprosy, and it wasn't possible for them to keep me on, working with food, once they knew that."

So after a few months of roaming from place to place—his health deteriorating as he went—he decided he needed to change his approach. "I thought, okay, now I am fed up with hotels, they are always sending me out, so I'll go and carry luggage and that kind of thing on the railway platforms instead. Otherwise I have to put up with people always pointing out that I have this big disease, even though there were no big signs: really only the thickening of my ear lobes and a few patches." And so it was that Chandra Prakash found himself working on Madras Central station, alongside the man he did not yet know was his brother, at the tail end of the 1970s.

Having shared their stories with one another, and having reminisced about the little time they had shared together as a family, back in Kumbakonam, they decided that Chandra Prakash should travel to Bombay to report to the family that they were both alive and, apart from having leprosy, were well and living in Madras. Das did not want to go directly himself. Even after all those years he still felt awkward about seeing Subrahmanyam again, having run away from both of the jobs he fixed him up with. The family was not aware that Das had leprosy, either, so he decided it would be best for his brother to break the news. Chandra Prakash confirmed the story: "I remember, my brother put me on the train to Bombay, and I went to their house in Chembur—I still remembered the address—and my big mother, Parvathi, answered the door. 'Who are you?' she said, and I told her, 'I am Chandra Prakash.' It had been a long time: I was only ten when she last saw me, and now I was nearly twenty. I was also much blacker than I had been then, my skin had been affected by the tablets. I told her I'd come from Madras, and she asked my father's name and my brother's name, just to check it was really me."

Chandra Prakash did not recall what his mother said or what she thought about the situation, nor what happened once he entered the house. He was vague about the kind of work he and Das did and avoided telling them that they were living on the pavement outside the station. His family, perhaps, avoided pressing too hard for details they did not want to hear. But they were all glad, he said, that he and his brother had been reunited and that he was going to get treatment now at the hospital in Madras for his leprosy. "And they reserved me a place on the train back a week later, and gave me money and other things—clothes, food items—to take with me for the pair of us. Subrahmanyam had just retired then, and they were all coming back within the year to Madras themselves—to build somewhere in Arumbakkam they said—so they told me that we should write and stay in touch and that they would visit us there when they returned."

Back in Madras, Chandra Prakash was well looked after by Das's friends. "Nobody was allowed to harm him, nor his friend, once they knew he was my brother. They loved him even more than they loved me! One day some shoemaker beat my brother—he didn't want him around near where he was working, something like that—and Manoj was furious about it. When he found out he took a horse whip to that cobbler. 'Why did you beat Iyer Chandra Prakash!' he had demanded, full of anger, and he hit him twice across the head with the whip. He cut his head open: there was blood everywhere and that man needed stitches, like the policeman had done. Nobody bothered Chandra Prakash after that!"

Chandra Prakash did need treatment though, and soon after he was admitted to the government hospital, where he stayed for more than a year. "He was full of leprosy reactions by then," Das remembered, "the disease was fully coming out over his body, and he was covered with boils. But they looked after him well there and we, from the station, all visited him often, and he started to get better." The fact that he was in the hospital also meant they had a suitable place for the reunion with their mother and Parvathi when, as good as their word, they arrived back in Madras a year later. They were staying in a rented house in Mandaveli while they oversaw the construction of a new, brick and concrete family home. "I didn't really want them to see everyone on the station," Das admitted. "I thought they might be upset to see how we were living, outside, and along with all those other station people. We hadn't told them we were working as porters. After that, once they'd seen Chandra Prakash was being looked after in hospital, I used to visit them, maybe once every two or three months, and when we left they'd always give us some money or some clothes and other things."

The reunion with his mother, like most of their meetings over the next few years, was mediated through Parvathi, the more talkative of the two women. "I'm sure she'd felt sorrow when we all left," Das said, "and that, even though she can't say it openly, she worried about us inside. Years later, she told me about how she once saw someone fall under a train and that, from a distance, he had looked like me. She had to go up close and peer over the platform to discover that it was someone else. And when she saw reports about accidents happening or bodies being found she'd have those thoughts again. Could those boys be my sons? Her eyes would show tears sometimes but she wouldn't say anything. It was too late by then: she'd lived with that other family longer than she had been with us, and they loved her very much. She's taken good care of them, looking after Parvathi and doing the cooking and cleaning in the house. I think those boys loved her more than their own mother."

The one piece missing now from their united family was Das and Chandra Prakash's father, Gajavakra, from whom no-one had heard word since he absconded from the meals hotel back in 1968. Although memories of his father were thin in his stories of growing up—mentions of him confined mostly to his departures at various key junctures—Das had clearly longed to see Gajavakra again for a long time. "I always kept my eyes peeled for him," he said. "I can remember one day waking up on the wall where we slept sometimes in the afternoon, and, sitting up, caught sight of this man walking along the road away from the station. He was the right size, the right age, everything. So I leapt down from the wall and starting chasing after him. 'Gajavakra Iyer! Gajavakra Iyer!' I shouted out. But he didn't respond or turn around, so I ran up to him and caught his arm. He turned around and I saw his face, close up, and he said that it wasn't him, that it wasn't Gajavakra." Das's face fell. "It upset me. I'd got my hopes up, and then they were dashed. I went back to the wall and cried for quite some time. But life had to go on. I kept on finding seats for people, carrying their luggage and taking them to hotels, sleeping, reading detective stories and playing cards. What else could I do?"

Next time, however, he was more certain. "I saw two men sitting there talking on the platform. One of them was my father. I hadn't seen him for fifteen years, but he hadn't changed that much since I last saw him. So I went over and sat nearby, and he looked around at me but he didn't recognize me straightaway. The last time he'd seen me I'd been a boy—sixteen or something. This was 1981, so I was about thirty-one, and I'd been working on the stations for a few years and my skin was darker from taking the leprosy drugs, so I'd changed more than he had. I went up to him, and—just so I could be sure—asked him who he was. He looked suspicious. 'Who are you to be asking me that?' he said sharply. So I told him. His jaw dropped open a little and he started to smile: 'This is my son!' he said to the other person with him, who was also a leprosy patient. 'You can leave me to talk to him now and I'll find you later on.'"

And that was it—the third and final cinematic moment that appears in all Das's accounts of his story. He took Gajavakra out of the station and across the road to the hospital to meet Chandra Prakash, where—"because Chandra Prakash was very popular with the staff and they all wanted to help him'— their father was able to bathe, eat a meal they brought him of curd rice and sambar, and sleep overnight. He was treated like a VIP. Word was sent, meanwhile, to Parvathi's place in Mandaveli, that they had finally met Gajavakra, and that they could also meet outside the hospital the next day, before Gajavakra caught his train.

"In the morning," said Das, "my father came back to see me outside the station. We took breakfast and he talked about how he was living now in his own place in a leprosy colony in coastal Andhra Pradesh, less than eight hours away from Madras on the train, and that I should come back there with him when he left that evening." As they were talking another leprosy patient approached Gajavakra. They exchanged pleasantries, and the other man asked him how "amma garu"—a respectful term for a woman—was getting on. Gajavakra had replied that she was very well. "I thought to myself, 'Who is amma garu?'" recalled Das, "but I didn't say anything. I thought, 'there's lots of time now. We can move slowly.'" Then, later that same afternoon, Parvathi and Subbalakshmi arrived, and the reunion was finally complete.

"There was no question of my father and mother moving back together," said Das. "They had been apart for too long. Even then, at that meeting, they didn't say much to each other. Just greetings and other things, and news about other members of the family. And most of that came from Parvathi; my mother just stood quietly by her side. It was emotional though. She told me to take care of my father, and said to my father that he should take care of Chandra Prakash and me. She was pleased that we had all found each other." Leprosy was not mentioned directly, but they all knew the role it had played in keeping them apart. Finally, after more tears and promises to stay in touch, Parvathi gave the men Rs1,000, and the two women took a rickshaw home. Das and Gajavakra—after saying goodbye to Chandra Prakash, who they left in the hospital—went to Egmore Station and caught the train to the town nearest to Anandapuram.

They arrived at around midnight. "After we got down on the platform, we took a flat cycle rickshaw down the dark lanes to the colony. It was very quiet then, more like our village than a place like Madras." In the 1980s, when electricity supply was still very limited, the night sky was much darker than it is today, and stars were far more visible. Das remembered: "A *dora-garu* [term of respect for a man—usually a foreigner], Solly, was standing by the roadside as we came into the colony. He greeted my father and my father told him that I was his son. He greeted me warmly. Eventually we got to my father's house and, because it was night, the door was bolted from the inside. He knocked, and I heard a woman's voice coming from inside. I remembered the conversation he'd had with the man at the station, the one who'd asked him how amma garu was, and then it clicked in my mind: ah, I thought, he's connected to someone else. This woman, who later was introduced as Elizabeth Rani, opened the door, and she couldn't see properly who was standing there with my father in the darkness. 'Shakara! Hello, is that you?' she shouted towards me—that was the name of one of their friends who lived in another leprosy colony and came to visit them sometimes—but my father explained to her, 'no, no, it's my son!' She was surprised but pleased. She opened her mouth wide and said: 'Aha! Nice, good! Come, come inside my son, come inside!' That's how I met Elizabeth Rani and came to learn my father had remarried. But I never asked him about it, and he never told me anything either."

By the time I was interviewing Das for his life story, Gajavakra was no longer around to account for his movements in the years after he absconded from the canteen in Madras. But between them Chandra Prakash and Das were able to fill me in with at least the basic details. Gajavakra's first stop after leaving Madras had been Paranur Government Leprosy Home, in Salem District, about thirty miles further south. It was not far from where he had worked on his previous trips away from home, so perhaps he already had contacts with the home there. Back when they all lived in Madras, he had always kept his leprosy hidden from the family. He received medical treatment for his leprosy, and worked as a cook. He stayed there, working and receiving treatment, for about a year, Das thought, and then shifted to another leprosy home in Attur, Salem District, nearly 150 miles further south. Quite why he moved there is uncertain: perhaps the treatment for his particular type of leprosy was more readily available there, or perhaps they had more places for patients. What *is* known, however, is that it was in Attur that he met Elizabeth Rani. Like Gajavakra, she was born a Brahmin in Tamil Nadu, and like him she also had leprosy. Beyond their caste, however, Elizabeth Rani had little in common with Gajavakra's first wife—at least by the time I met both women in the late 1980s and 1990s. Elizabeth Rani was as loud and as forceful in manner as Subbalakshmi was quiet and timid; and while Subbalakshmi was a slight woman who seemed to slip almost unnoticed into the background, Elizabeth Rani's bright sarees, jangling rows of bangles, gold earrings and extravagant bunches of fragrant jasmine in her hair ensured that her presence was felt. She was frequently at the centre of fights, and no one could accuse her of not being able to hold her own. Their wedding had been of the informal variety, made by Gajavakra tying a *mangala sutram*—marriage string—around Elizabeth Rani's neck, and marking the event with a small tea party.

From there, eventually, the couple traveled together to another leprosy colony in Nellore, across the border in Andhra Pradesh, although there may have been other leprosy colonies along the way. In the Nellore colony, which was funded by the Catholic church in Rome and run by the local Bishop, they converted to Catholicism, and received a monthly ration of food and other provisions. "It was apparently very strict there," said Das. "You received your monthly ration, had jobs to do for which you got some kind of allowance, and you were not allowed to go out—even for just a couple of days—without permission." While they were living there, either he or Elizabeth Rani came to visit the mission hospital close to Anandapuram for treatment that was not available at the time in Nellore. "When he was there," said Das, "he visited the leprosy colony next door while one of them was admitted to the hospital and treatment, and realized that it was a convenient place to stay. There was no ration of food, but you could come and go as you pleased. Since they needed to stay near the hospital while one of them underwent a long course of treatment, they decided to join this colony—Anandapuram—and to build themselves a mud and thatch house there."

It was to this house, four years later, that Gajavakra took his son.

NOTES

1. This strategy of moving through space as well as time in our interviews was inspired, in part, by earlier reading of de Certeau's influential essay, "Walking in the City" in Michel de Certeau, *The Practice of Everyday Life* (Berkeley: University of California Press, 1984), 102–118.

2. See, for a focus on friendship as an alternative to anthropology's traditional focus on kinship, Amit Desai and Evan Killick, eds., *The Ways of Friendship: Anthropological Perspectives* (Oxford: Berghahn, 2010), and, for a specifically Indian example—which resonates with Das's own descriptions of his significant relationships—Peggy Froerer, "Close Friends: The Importance of Proximity in the Formation of Friendship in Chhattisgarh, India," in *The Ways of Friendship: Anthropological Perspectives*, eds Amit Desai and Evan Killick, (Oxford: Berghahn, 2010), 133–153.

3. There is a fairly long history of studies of gambling in South Asia—for example, see John A. Price, "Gambling in Traditional Asia," *Anthropologica* (NS) 14, 2 (1972): 157–180. On gambling in anthropology more generally, an obvious starting point is Clifford Geertz, "Deep Play: Notes on the Balinese Cockfight," *Daedalus* 101, 1 (1972): 1–37. A more recent example—on horse racing in particular—is Rebecca Cassidy, *The Sport of Kings: Kinship, Class and Thoroughbred Breeding in Haymarket* (Cambridge: Cambridge University Press, 2002).

4. Perhaps the richest ethnographic account of the Emergency can be found in Emma Tarlo, *Unsettling Memories: Narratives of the Emergency in India* (Berkeley, University of California Press: 2003). There was also a plethora of work published in the immediate aftermath, including, for example, Michael Henderson, *Experiment with untruth: India under Emergency* (Delhi: Macmillan, 1977); P. N. Dhar, *Indira Gandhi, the "Emergency" and Indian Democracy* (New Delhi: Oxford University Press, 2000); Brij Mohan Toofan, *When Freedom*

Bleeds: Journey through Indian Emergency (Delhi: Ajanta Publications, 1988). My own interest in the era had originally been piqued by references in novels to the era—many of which offered more sensationalized accounts of events against which I inevitably read Das's personal accounts—such as Rohinton Mistry, *A Fine Balance* (London: Faber and Faber, 1996). More generally on Indira Gandhi, see, for example, Katherine Frank, *Indira: The Life of Indira Nehru Gandhi* (London: Harper Collins, 2010).

5. The sterilisation programme spawned much fiction, including, again, Mistry, *A Fine Balance*. See also Frank, *Indira: The Life of Indira Nehru Gandhi*, and Pai Panandiker, *Family planning under the Emergency: policy implications and incentives and disincentives* (New Delhi: Radiant Publishers, 1978).

Chapter Five

Anandapuram

Das did not stay long in Anandapuram, at least not on that first visit in 1981. He was pleased that he had been reunited with his father and, having also made contact again with his mother and his brother, felt more anchored in the world than he had done for a long time. He was no longer on his own. But for someone who had wandered free for more than a decade, a move back to family life in the countryside was too much to contemplate. He spent a couple of days there, getting to know Elizabeth Rani and Timothy—as Gaja-vakra had been renamed by the priest when he converted to Catholicism—and then headed back to Madras. His brother was, in any case, still in the hospital, and he needed Das to look after him.

Anandapuram, the village where most of my interviews with Das for this book took place, on a verandah not one hundred yards from where Elizabeth Rani still lived, was a very different place in the early 1980s to the one it had developed into by the new century. Back then, many of the houses were still mud huts: small circular rooms topped with conical overhanging roofs of bamboo and straw. They kept out the heat in the hot summers, but they offered only the most basic protection against the rest of the elements, and were particularly ill-equipped to withstand the cyclonic storms to which the area was prone. Even the more substantial houses—like the three-roomed place occupied by an English nurse who had recently come to live and work in the village—were constructed from mud and thatch. And although there was an electricity supply by then, the current—when it was not off altogether—was often too weak to light a bulb sufficiently to read by.

People had started settling there, as I already knew off pat from my previous trips to work and conduct research in the community, in the late 1950s. Like Timothy and Elizabeth Rani they had moved there, either on to what was then a patch of railway-owned scrubland adjacent to the Mission hospital, where they simply squatted, or to plots continuous with it that they purchased from a local cashew nut farmer.

According to a doctor I interviewed who had worked in the hospital, the flight from the hospital's compound, enclosed, as it was, by a ten-foot wall, came about with a change in disease control. Until the late 1950s, patients had lived there in their own family units, receiving uncooked food rations from which they prepared meals for themselves. The management of the hospital, however, had observed that people were cooking and burning their hands where they had no sensation, and were becoming increasingly impaired as a result. In response to this, they decided that food should instead be cooked and served centrally, rather than by the patients themselves, and that the patients should stay in wards, not in family units. For those who had married or had children during their stay at the hospital, this was not a popular option, and many of them left to set up what became Anandapuram Colony.

In addition, some patients, now that leprosy was recognized as curable, were discharged after many years of institutionalization. As was the case for Timothy, it was too late to return to an earlier life, especially as the route Timothy had followed—re-marriage to a fellow patient and conversion to Christianity—was a very common one. And if leprosy had meant a severing of links with what was once home, a return there ten years later and picking up where one had left off was not a viable option.

Trees and wild plants were cleared to make way for individual houses, for a makeshift church—also built from mud and palm leaf thatch in its original incarnation—and, initially, for a single well from which they could draw water. Life was tough there, especially in the beginning, but, for those who chose it, it was considered preferable to the controls imposed upon them and their movements if they stayed within the hospital environment.

Here, in Anandapuram, they were free. That meant they could go begging, an activity that was more than frowned upon in the hospital, and have some control over their own income and expenditure. Free rations of basic provisions were all very well, but there was little scope within the hospital, unless they were able to secure jobs there, to raise money beyond them. Even in Anandapuram, there was not much possibility beyond begging. A few entrepreneurs brought in extra rupees by setting up petty shops and tea stalls, and a few made money from smuggling ration rice across state borders and selling it on the black market at a profit. For most people, though, begging was seen as the only plausible option. Employment prospects, for leprosy disfigured people who were both uneducated and institutionalized, were not especially high.

Begging was initially an activity that settlers carried out on their own or in couples, but it soon developed into a collective occupation, conducted by what were known as *zanda* [flag] groups.[1] They were so-called because fiftccn or twenty people would group together under a single large *zanda*, carried on poles at either end by two members of the group, which explained who they were and why they were begging. They reminded me of the big cloth banners brought out by trade unions and other protest groups during marches, and were used to similar effect: to draw attention to their cause. The rest of the group either played drums, horns, rattles or tambourines, or they carried simple collection tins, fashioned out of old cans topped with cloth, in which slits had been cut for donations to pass through. Donors were thus spared direct physical contact with those affected by leprosy. It proved more lucrative, and safer, than begging alone, particularly when—as happened later, in the 1970s—*zanda* groups started going as far a field as Madras, Calcutta and Bombay, and even to Assam, Rajasthan and Nagaland. By then the groups were smaller—typically eight or nine members—and were organized under the control of a *zanda maistry*, who took a bigger cut of the profits. These groups would stay, sleeping rough, in their chosen locations for forty days or more, only returning briefly to the colony to deposit money with their other family members. Both Timothy and Elizabeth Rani had been involved in these begging groups since joining the colony. Timothy had been returning from one such trip, in Madras, when Das had seen him on the station. "They were open about it with Chandra Prakash and me," Das said, "and we didn't think much about it. They were leprosy patients living in a leprosy colony, and that's how most people living there made their money. It was just how it was. But we didn't ever tell my mother that: I think we just said he did some kind of work in a leprosy hospital. Cooking, probably. We never told her that he had married someone else either, and if she ever found out or suspected, she never mentioned it to us." Begging, in some ways, remained more taboo than leprosy itself, and I still know families of all castes who, despite having brought their wider kin around to the fact that they have been affected by leprosy, continue to protect them from the knowledge that they also go begging. Although Das was proud of the fact that he had never personally succumbed to begging, he admits that some of the work he was doing on the station was not so very far removed. It was "a platform life," as he described it.

By the mid-1960s, the colony's settlers had also registered themselves as an Association under the Societies' Act, with the aim of raising funds from the government for medicines—to be sent directly to them rather than via the hospital, with which relations had become strained—and other welfare benefits. The son of a local Congress party councillor helped them with the registration, in so doing also getting Anandapuram's residents registered to vote and laying the foundations of a longstanding affinity with the Congress Party. Under the rules of the new Association, there were seven elected male Elders, general body meetings and membership fees, initially of Rs0.25 per member. By the time Timothy and Elizabeth Rani joined it had risen to around Rs7, but it was worth it to have a place of their own and the opportunity to make a living, even if it was from begging.

Timothy's arrival, in around 1977, pre-dated, although only just, the arrival of foreigners in the village. They had become well-established by the time he took Das there in 1981. It was also with the arrival of foreigners that formal records started to be kept in English—especially fundraising newsletters and pamphlets to send back to their contacts in the West. This kind of documentation is, of course, necessarily highly partial, and it also filtered back into the community's ideas about itself. Villagers learned about their own recent history by reading or being told outsiders' accounts of it. I remember one occasion when, having asked someone about the history of their community, they responded in oddly familiar terms. I later discovered that the story matched, almost word for word, an account I had written up several years earlier for a fundraising pamphlet, which, in turn, had been spun from earlier pamphlets and memories of those working in the office at the time. My words, written without much care for history but with the intention of appealing to potential overseas donors, had became part of official colony history.[2]

Nevertheless, the files and documents that started to accumulate at around that time—many of which now sit gathering thick layers of dust and sustaining termites on sagging shelves in the community's office—offered me a rich source of material to compare against people's oral accounts of how the village developed, most of which were collected not via interviews, which tended to lead to formulaic accounts, internalized through repetition of the messages contained in those yellowing pamphlets at public events, but through general conversations that took place more naturally over more than a year's fieldwork.

Although the details are contested depending on who is telling the story, all agree that Brother Jack, then in his mid-thirties, was the first of the long-stay foreigners to arrive in 1979. He had been a small town businessman from the American mid-west and, like many westerners who arrived in the 1960s and 1970s, claimed he had headed to India for spiritual enlightenment. I never met him, and only ever saw one photograph of him; a slightly fuzzy black and white print, which offered only a general impression of what he looked like. A thick beard, long dark hair and large tinted spectacles hid most of his facial features. He was dressed entirely in white. Someone once said that he resembled Jesus; maybe that was part of his attraction. On the day he arrived in Anandapuram, he was on the way to an ashram in Kerala, on part of a five-month pilgrimage he had undertaken after, he claimed, renouncing all worldly possessions and receiving his Sanyasi initiation. He had, runs the story, stopped off in a nearby town, and someone he knew there introduced him to the village. Something about the resilience of the people, and the fact that they were receiving no outside support at all at that time, clearly impressed him, because he returned in 1980 and asked the Elders if he could settle there. He was, he claimed, following a calling from Jesus Christ. The Elders agreed, and developments that were gradually taking place in the village were accelerated.

Brother Jack, as he modelled himself, lived simply in one of the round huts typical of the village, set up a makeshift office, and started to canvass his contacts for funds. A small clinic was the first priority, followed by a series of rehabilitation projects that were intended to provide an alternative to begging. The weaving and stitching of bags and table linen is the main one that has survived and the only one that everyone remembers, although the records are replete with schemes, from silk-production (aborted after the mulberry bushes, grown to feed the silk worms, withered in the intense heat of the summer), to goat rearing (they suffered badly from worms and other conditions). Later came mushroom farming, rabbits, chickens and dairy buffaloes, photo frame production, plastics moulding and a synthetic gem cutting unit. Some income was generated, and those involved learned new skills, but most of the schemes eventually foundered without subsidies, and none—apart from the weaving and tailoring—offered tenable long-term alternatives to begging. The latter was simply too lucrative by comparison. Those who did work—and those who were unable either to work or beg—ate together with Jack and those who followed him there in a larger round hut that was constructed for the purpose.

The flurry of activity in the early 1980s, and the charm and energy for which Jack was renowned, was also a pull for other foreigners who wanted to help. He put Anandapuram on the map. Solly, the man on the road who had greeted Das on his first visit, was one of the longer term visitors. He had been roped in to help with the accounts. Originally a Jewish accountant from London he had the skills that were required, even though he had not used them for the best part of twenty years, and was much keener on devoting his energies to spiritual matters. Solly was forty-seven when he came to Anandapuram after meeting Jack in an ashram a year or two earlier. He had converted to Roman Catholicism in 1968 by way of Buddhism, and still spent as many hours of the day as he could in the religious meditation he had learned as part of that earlier faith. Meditation, he once told me, was his main work; the accounts were something he had to do inbetween. I never saw Solly dressed in anything other than loose white pyjams and short white kurta—a suit of which he kept just two sets—and he wore thick, horn-rimmed spectacles.

Emma Cox, a twenty-six-year-old British nurse, also came to live in Anandapuram in 1981. She knew many of the residents from when they had lived in the hospital, where she had worked as a nurse since 1978, and was attracted by the work going on in Anandapuram. She crossed the railway line along with Narasingha Naidu, a patient who had first become her night watchman and then her friend and Telugu teacher, and his young bride-to-be Rajamani. The three-roomed house they occupied became a centre point for shorter-stay visitors over the years that followed, who congregated there for meals and to celebrate festivals.

Das, meanwhile, continued his life on Madras Central Station, and Chandra Prakash continued to recover in hospital. But by the time he was released, fully cured, in 1982, the station held no enduring attractions for him. As both of them had pointed out to me, unlike Das he was ill-suited to a porter's work, and was far too timid to prosper from touting hotel rooms and other services. Consequently, Chandra Prakash went straight to Anandapuram Colony, where, like Das, he became a member, and, unlike Das, stayed there with his father and step-mother.

"They were going for *zanda* groups, so I went with them," Chandra Prakash recalled. "My first trip was in December 1983, I think, when we went to Calcutta. Kotta Krishna was the *maistry*, and my father asked him if I could join them too. He and Elizabeth Rani carried the collection tins and, because I had good hands, I was given the drums to play. There were eight of us in total." He continued with that work for the next four years, until his marriage was arranged in 1987. Before that, however, came Das's decision—under pressure from his father—finally to settle in Anandapuram. Despite all that had happened to them, Timothy was still keen that his sons should marry in the right order, and that meant finding a match for Das before Chandra Prakash could be settled.

Das remembers returning to Anandapuram for the New Year celebrations at the end of 1984. It was a time of major upheaval in India, following the assassination of the prime minister, Indira Gandhi, by her Sikh body guards in October. In the immediate aftermath, more than one thousand Sikhs were killed by rioters out to avenge the death of their leader.[3] On the main road that ran past the Mission hospital—opposite the spot where Anandapuram villagers hailed cycle rickshaws into the local town—a giant cut-out of Gandhi, perhaps twenty-feet tall, loomed over passers-by. Two smaller images of turbaned Sikh men were depicted firing their weapons up at her, a stream of crimson blood exuding from the prime minister's body. Although feelings were running high, however, in the South there were far fewer Sikhs for other communities to vent their anger on, and Indira's Congress Party—pitched against local parties of the southern states—was less idolized than in other parts of India. In Anandapuram, men in the teashops read the newspapers and shook their heads in dismay at the horrors that were unfolding, but the politics of Delhi were a long way off. It was perhaps for this reason that the assassination never came up in Das's account. Perhaps he thought it was such an internationally-recognized event that it scarcely warranted mention in his own biography. Or perhaps it was because Das was more focused on the feeling that his time at Madras Central Station was about to come to an end.

Timothy had come to the station in Madras for him earlier in December: "He didn't press me then to come and live in Anandapuram," says Das, "although I knew that's what he really wanted. But he just said, 'Come for the festival at least, then we can see.'" The new year festival is big in Anandapuram and was celebrated with more fanfare than Christmas because those away begging in *zanda* groups all returned to the village for it. The sanyasi had left the village to pursue other projects by then, and Emma had replaced him as administrator of the colony. The overseas volunteers kept coming, however, and it was in that guise that I first arrived, in August 1984. It was not long after the Indian army stormed the Golden Temple in Amritsar, in a bid to flush out the Sikh separatists who were taking refuge there; an event that prefigured Gandhi's assassination a few months later.[4] It was also just days after the national government had backed a coup which removed—for a time—Andhra's chief minister, who was replaced with one favored by the Congress Party. It was in protest at this that the train I was travelling on from Bombay to Anandapuram was halted and stoned by protestors who had laid down on the tracks in front of it. To me, at the time, being woken up by the sound of rocks and sticks rebounding from the train was just part of the excitement of being in India, a new and apparently fantastically different place. For all I knew at the time, this was an everyday occurrence. In retrospect, it was a sign of how volatile Indian politics were at that time.

Although my memories of that first trip to Anandapuram have become merged with a range of recollections from across the ensuing years, I remember the communal new year celebratory meal—held at lunchtime on January 1, 1985—very well. There were two parallel lines of mats stretched out across the empty expanse of sand in front of the school, maybe one hundred metres long in total. If you were sitting in the middle, as I was, it was hard to make out who was sitting at either end. Men were placed on one side and women on the other with disposable leaf plates laid out in front of them. The servers, bearing aluminium basins of rice or vats of dhal, pickles, vegetable curries, poppadoms and curd, ran up and down the space inbetween the two lines of mats, responding to our demands for more. Once sated, diners indicated they had finished by folding over their leaf plates and walking over to the water pot to wash their hands. Servers removed the used plates, and other diners would take their places until everyone, maybe 700 of us, had eaten. The skies were blue and it was a bright, sunny day, but, this being the winter, it was not excessively hot.

Das was present at that meal, too, although I did not meet him then. The first sighting of him I can remember, a month or so later, was when his father brought him to the office to press Emma to give him some sort of work. Even then, I only saw him through the bamboo struts that connected the low mud wall of the office to the palm leaf conical roof above. Timothy left him outside while he came in to make Das's case. He was, Timothy told Emma, thirty-five-years-old, had a secondary school education, good English and an ability with numbers. He had been working on Madras Central Railway station as an unofficial porter because his leprosy debarred him from other forms of employment, but if he could be given an alternative job in Anandapuram he would be able to stay on and get married. Without work, said Timothy, it would be difficult to keep him there with his family.

I cannot remember, now, the ins and outs of Emma and Timothy's exchange, although Das recalls a general promise that she would do what she could to find him something. "Once I was there in Anandapuram, my father had said to me, 'At least write an application to the office for a job. Then, if you get one, you can stay on here with us. Your brother's already here, so we'd all be together.' So I thought, okay, why not?"

The other part of Timothy's plan was to get Das married. He and Elizabeth Rani had mooted marriage in the past. There had even been a couple of tentative proposals, and they had never ceased their search for a suitable bride. Until now, however, he had been able to shrug off their suggestions. "I wasn't interested," Das said. "I'd decided a long time before that I didn't want to marry, and I'd even had that family planning operation, so I didn't expect it ever to happen. It was only after coming here to Anandapuram, and seeing all these leprosy patients who had got married and had children, that I realized it was some kind of possibility."

Even on this occasion, had Timothy told Das why they were going to another leprosy colony in Khammam, around one hundred miles north-west of Anandapuram, he might have tried to get out of it. But Timothy did not reveal his plans: he just said that they were going to visit some friends of his, and Das, who never liked staying still, was happy to go along for the ride. "He took me with him on the train along with Koteswara, who was one of the Elders then and whose wife came from that place, and we went to this house, where they brought out this girl called Mariya. She was very small, thin and young. Her father, it was her step-father, actually, he introduced her to my father as his daughter, and my father introduced me as his son. Then I started to understand, even though I couldn't understand Telugu, which is what they were speaking to each other in, that they were talking about marrying us to each other. I couldn't say anything, not in front of the families, and not without the language, so I just sat there quietly and waited."

Koteswara, the Elder and a good friend of Timothy's, had set up the meeting. Brokering marriages between leprosy colonies was, and remains, one of the Elders' most useful functions. In this case, he had told Timothy that there was a healthy girl at the Khammam colony from a very poor family ready for marriage, and he had told Mariya's family about Das. Mariya's family was not Brahmin, or anything close. They were Madigas, or cobbler caste: one of the two main scheduled—formerly untouchable—castes in Andhra. Das's family would not otherwise have considered marrying into a lower caste, but leprosy and Christian conversion, while they did not elide caste entirely, did make it less significant in terms of marital alliances. And finding a Brahmin wife for a thirty-five-year-old leprosy-affected man who had spent the last sixteen years of his life on the streets would have been a tall order, particularly as Timothy was in a rush to organize a union before Das upped and left them for Madras again.

Mariya was only thirteen or fourteen. Embodying her poverty, she was also physically tiny. She has the narrowest shoulders I think I have ever seen on a grown woman, scarcely wider than her head. Although she was young, Mariya was on the verge of puberty and, as was the case for many families, her parents were keen to marry her before any rumors about her sleeping with boys—which were common, however much girls kept themselves to themselves—could begin to circulate and spoil her reputation. Finding respectable partners for girls from poor families who could not afford even a modest dowry, especially when there was also leprosy in the family, was never easy. If the girl got a bad name it became even harder.

Guruswamy, Mariya's step-father, was her mother's third husband. The first, a bicycle mechanic, had died after fathering Balakrishna, who eventually took up cycle repairs himself. The second husband, Venkatasubbaiah, was the father of both Mariya and her younger brother Venkanna. Tired of his excessive drinking and physical violence, Mariya's mother had left him, taking the children with her, for Guruswamy. Both of them had taken treatment for leprosy, and, from their base in the Khammam leprosy colony, had gone begging together, taking the children to sleep alongside them on the pavement. "The way she was, it was difficult for Mariya's mother to be a good example to her children," said Das. "She was a patient, she didn't do any work, and didn't send any of them to school. Mariya used to get left to look after the youngest son."

A week after the visit to Khammam, however, word came back from Mariya's family that they were not interested in pursuing the marriage. Das was not told. "If I had been," he said, "I'd have told to my father, 'Don't press unnecessarily! If she doesn't want to marry then let's not marry.' We should just have left it." Elizabeth Rani, however, was not a woman for leaving things. She went straight off to Khammam herself, accompanied by Komati Ramulu, a village chit fund manager and money-lender, to help seal the arrangement.

There were two main problems. The first, Mariya's parents said, was that they had no money, not even to cover the basics. Her mother's husband, Guruswamy, was old, disabled, and without much source of income. The second problem was that Mariya was not happy about marrying a man around twenty years her senior. Her step-father had dealt with the latter issue

himself, by using the not uncommon strategy of taking an overdose of pre-
scription medicines—in his case, the leprosy drug Dapsone—in order to
convince her. "First you agreed to this, and now you try to back out of it!" he
apparently shouted at her, before theatrically and publicly cramming his
mouth with Dapsone tablets and downing them with a glass of water. Gen-
dered hysteria ensued—the women of the family wailing and the men shouting—and Guruswamy, once he had been forced to vomit back the pills, was
ultimately unharmed. Mariya, however, was left with no choice but to concede to their plans. Marriage to a man more than twice her age must have
seemed preferable to living with the blame for her step-father's untimely
demise.⁵

The second problem, that of money, was resolved more straightforwardly
by Elizabeth Rani. Das reported: "My step-mother told them, okay, if you've
got no money, if that's what the problem is, we'll give Rs1,000 for saris and
other ornaments necessary for the marriage, and we'll cover everything else.
Somehow they agreed, and Elizabeth Rani borrowed the money from Komati
Ramulu."

There were prayer meetings already scheduled to take place in Khammam
on 21st, 22nd and 23rd February, so it was decided that the marriage would
be held there. The day before Das's family set off, the call came from the
colony's office. I had already left India, a few days earlier, but Emma,
Daniel, the accounts clerk, and the office typist, Indira, were all there. "They
told me that I needed to go house-to-house in the village, and gather together
some data," Das remembered. "I needed to get names, ages and details about
what they had done previously, before they had leprosy and came to live
there. 'If you do that,' Emma said, 'we'll give you a small weekly allowance,
and your meals will be provided.' I knew my father really wanted me to stay,
so I said, okay, let's give it a try. I had to start work on February 25th."

Before that, he had his marriage to attend to, and, prior to that, his baptism. "Just before the wedding, which was on 23rd, Mariya and I and several
others were taken by the pastor down to the canal, where he did a Bible
reading. Then we all had our heads dunked three times under the water, and
he said to me, 'Now your name is . . .'—and he paused while he thought of
one—'. . . Jobdas!' That's how it was done, your new Christian name would
be selected on the spot. Or sometimes the pastor would open the Bible and
give you the first name he saw there."

A religious conversion, it seemed to me, was almost as big a deal—
perhaps an even bigger one—than getting married and starting a new life in a
new village in a new state: especially for a Tamil Brahmin whose brother had
spent much of his childhood learning mantras and how to officiate over
Hindu ceremonies. But Das shrugged when I asked him about it. "There was
no other choice," he said simply. "In this colony, if you want to stay here and
get married, these were the customs that are followed. If I'd taken her to get

married in my uncle's house, then it would have been a Hindu wedding. But we're not thinking about it in that way. We are thinking, we want to get married, and we do it according to the local custom. And I already knew that my father had become a Catholic when he was in Nellore, so this was not a big surprise." Religion, for all but the most devoted core, was as much about practice and expectation as it was about absolute belief, although, as Das himself had pointed out to me, the former was also inextricably linked to the latter.[6]

The marriage ceremony itself took place beneath the open-sided marquee that had been set up for the prayer meetings, and at the same time as three other weddings. "The other couples were all second marriages," Das said, "leprosy patients who had split up with their partners after getting the disease. The men were all my age or a bit older, but Mariya was the youngest of all the women there. She was just a girl."

"The ceremony was carried out by a Pastor from Ongole. They told us they'd give us a marriage certificate, but there was some complication about it because the pastor was registered in Ongole, and this was in a different district. It never came. But I thought, who needs a certificate? If we think we are married then we are. I wasn't interested in any of that, nor in having a big meeting and a big fuss. As long as the *mangala sutram* got tied around her neck that was all that mattered."

Unlike many of the marriages I attended in Anandapuram, where the family would feed the entire village in a feast not unlike the one which took place on January 1, numbers at Das's wedding were restricted to around 150 people—most of them relatives and neighbors of Mariya's family, and a dozen or so who had travelled there with Timothy and Elizabeth Rani from Anandapuram. "We just provided some pulao rice, some pappu charu [a thin lentil curry] and, I think, some mutton," said Das—relegating the meat component, which would have been the most important item to their Christian guests, to the end of his list. "I didn't eat it, so it was okay," he clarified, concerned that I would suspect him of eating the one thing he had always avoided, whatever the circumstances. "This was just the usual marriage food that people had to offer, it was just what the caterers prepared." Cost of the food, around Rs5,000, was also met by Timothy, who increased his loans with Komati Ramulu. He had also cashed in his chit funds, a popular way of saving money in Anandapuram.

I was never able to get fully to grips with how chit fund schemes worked, but, according to Das, they were very straightforward. "A group of people, say twenty, would agree to pay a set amount to a fund—let's say Rs100— every month for twenty-one months: a month for each member plus one for the chit fund manager. That means, each month there's a pot of Rs2,000. Whoever wants to draw that money has to bid for it, and those who need it most will usually bid the highest. So if I bid Rs200 for the money and win the bid, I'll take the Rs2,000, less my bid, which goes back into the pot. So, next month, there will be Rs2,000 plus Rs200—Rs2,200 in the pot. And the bidding starts again. The man who waits longest gets the most benefit."

The main beneficiary, though, is the chit fund manager, who also gets to bid for a share of the money without having to pay any in. These managers generally need to have some assets to start with—so that members trust them enough to pay out at the end of each month—but if they run a number of funds at the same time, they can generate a lot of money. For those less well placed and with major unavoidable expenditure—like weddings—being part of a chit fund is not quite so lucrative, especially when people have to bid hard on one chit fund only so they can get the money together to pay their dues on others. Komati Ramulu, who also ran a tea stall and breakfast food shop—serving dosas and idlis in the early mornings—was able to make a good profit.

The marriage and dinner over, Das was in a hurry to get back to Anandapuram, where he was due to start work two days later, on February 25. There was some more "lecturing"—as he referred to it as—from pastors and those giving testimony, and then the family returned to Anandapuram on the Krishna Express. Das and Mariya had hardly had a chance to look at one another, let alone speak very much, but the train home was crowded and, in any case, they had no common language. Although Das was fluent or good in Tamil, English, Hindi and Marathi, he had yet to master Telugu, the only language Mariya knew. "I asked how she was, if everything was okay, but that was all," said Das, "and she was very shy. She just nodded and kept her head down." They took a cycle rickshaw from the station to the house and, once there, some of the neighbors came by to look at the new bride who had been brought back to the village. "She was afraid, that first week or so," said Das, "but my step-mother and my father could speak to her in Telugu, and her own mother arrived to stay a few days later, so she began to settle in."

Das's mind was anyway occupied with other things. He turned up at the office for duty on the Monday morning as planned, and was despatched around the village to carry out the survey he had been recruited for. It was, as he found out later, for getting together the information they needed to apply for funds for the old people from the charity Help the Aged. "They wanted me because I could write down and record the answers in English," he said, "and even I could manage in Telugu to ask someone their name." Being out, walking around and communicating with people was also the kind of work that Das liked. As long as he was on the move and constantly occupied, as he had been on the station, he was happy. The radical change in his living circumstances, although he had avoided it for as long as possible, did not seem so bad after all.

"I completed the survey in just four days, and then I was sitting in the office, going through the material I'd gathered, and Daniel and Emma were both trying to tally the accounts and not being able to," he said. "They'd been trying for weeks to get the numbers to add up and they just couldn't. Every time they tried, different numbers were coming out, and they were getting very frustrated with it. Daniel's family was from Tamil Nadu too—they were Kshatriyas—and so we'd been speaking together in Tamil. 'Here, let me take a look,' I said, and they were happy to let me have a go. I went through and I discovered that they weren't including the advances—the money people had taken out for purchases but hadn't yet returned—in their totals. It was a simple thing but nobody had found it until then. The amount missing in their calculations was equal to the money that people still had out in these advances. I had solved the problem."

Emma was impressed. Since Solly had left the colony four months earlier, managing the colony's accounts had been a major problem. A trained nurse who was now getting to grips with administration, double-entry book keeping was not a skill she was especially desperate to acquire. Reuben, an outside man they had recruited from the neighbouring town, with a degree in Commerce, had not been able to grasp the intricacies of the system either, and his assistant, Daniel, was only waiting for the opportunity to train as a lab technician. "Reuben stopped coming at around that time, I think," said Das, "and Daniel got his training in March that year, so I ended up staying on in the office and helping to look after the accounts. Having run a card school in Bombay, and from going to place bets on the horses in Madras, I'd had a lot of practice with numbers!"

Back at home, Mariya was slowly learning to fit in. It must have been hard with five of them—including Chandra Prakash—in their small house, one room with a covered verandah, but the climate was such that most of the living, including cooking and sleeping, took place in the open air. Elizabeth Rani was busy teaching Mariya to do things, Das told me. "She wasn't threatening her or shouting at her, not in those days. She'd just show her, and explain that things had to be done in a certain way because this was a Brahmin house, not a low caste one like the one she had come from. My brother, he also taught her how to cook, something he was very good at, from when he had worked in the hotels. He could make those delicious Tamil specialities like *vada* in curd that no-one else in the village could prepare properly. And I was also picking up Telugu—I was used to learning new languages, no?—and so, within a month or two we could communicate more freely."

There was also the matter of consummating the marriage, an event for which arrangements are specifically made. "After she'd been with us for about a month," said Das, "it was time to go for the 'first night.' My stepmother, and probably her mother too, had told her what to expect, and the room had been prepared especially for us. They had left sweetmeats in the room and had covered the bed with jasmine buds. But even though she'd been warned, she was very young and didn't have any kind of experience before that. She was a newly matured young girl and I was thirty-five, and I had experience, so it was difficult. When I went to touch her she moved away, and then she was shouting and screaming. She was terrified, and I didn't want to force her. Elizabeth Rani came and told her to be quiet and not to worry about it, that it was normal, but I thought it was better to leave it. I left her alone, and we just slept. Only gradually did she become convinced that this was something we should do, maybe after talking about it to other women she got to know. I think they share their experiences of their husbands, no?!"

Although Das was bemused by his new wife, life in the village otherwise seemed okay to him, and, after his years on the station platforms, he began to settle in. "I had the work in the office, and that gave me some respect," he said, "and life is going on. The only thing with Mariya was that she didn't know very much, and I needed to adjust to her. That was all. Otherwise she seemed to be all right: she was young, not educated, and not brought up in the proper way, I don't think, but these were problems that could be dealt with."

"Back then, I only got Rs1,100 a month salary, but I had no chit funds or loans to repay, and my father brought in enough money from begging to cover all the family's other needs. We didn't have children, or a television or the expense of going to the cinema: the films were in Telugu, and so I didn't have a lot of interest in seeing those films. And I hadn't made many friends in the colony at the time, so I hadn't got into the habit of playing cards or other things. Life seemed to be good."

NOTES

1. Staples, "Leprosy and Alms collecting in Mumbai."
2. James Staples and Katherine Smith, "Introduction," in *Extraordinary Encounters*.
3. Frank, *Indira*; Ritu Sarin, *The Assassination of Indira Gandhi* (New Delhi: Penguin Books, 1990).
4. See, for example, Robert L. Hardgrave Jr and Stanley A. Kochanek, *India: Government and Politics in a Developing Nation* (Boston: Thompson Wadsworth, 2008), 176–177; Joyce Pettigrew, "Take Not Arms Against Thy Sovereign: The Present Punjab Crisis and the Storming of the Golden Temple," *South Asia Research* 4, 2 (1984): 102; Gurharpal Singh, "Understanding the 'Punjab Problem,'" *Asian Survey* 27, 12 (1987):1268–1277; Frank, *Indira*; Sarin, *The Assassination of Indira Gandhi.*
5. As discussed in my research on suicide-related behaviours in India, such displays of death making and self-harm are far from isolated incidents. See, for example, James Staples, "The suicide niche: accounting for self-harm in a South Indian leprosy colony," in *Suicide in South Asia: Ethnographic Perspectives*, ed. James Staples. Special Issue of *Contributions to Indian Sociology* 46, 1–2 (2012): 117–144; James Staples, "Ethnographies of Suicide in South Asia." In *Suicide in South Asia: Ethnographic Perspectives*, ed. James Staples. Special Issue of

Contributions to Indian Sociology 46, 1–2 (2012): 1–28; and James Staples and Tom Widger, "Situating Suicide as an Anthropological Problem: Ethnographic Approaches to Understanding Self-Harm and Self-Inflicted Death," *Culture, Medicine and Psychiatry* 36, 2 (2012) 183–203.

6. James Staples, "Putting Indian Christianities into context: biographies of Christian conversion in a leprosy colony," *Modern Asian Studies* (2014, online); Geoffrey Oddie, *Hindu and Christian in South-East India* (London: Curzon Press, 1991).

Chapter Six

Good Times

Good times in Anandapuram continued, at least for the next five years. "When I think about all those years on the station," Das said, "my memories are of having an enjoyable time and gaining good experience, but they were also wasted years. Coming here, to this village, I saw families and children and realized that there was the possibility of having a normal life, even if you were a leprosy patient." Das was also in his mid-thirties by now, and that, he said, made a difference: "Working and living on the platform is easy enough when you're young and reasonably fit, but it gets harder as you get older. Coming here also meant I could have a rest."

The rosy quality that seems to tint Das's descriptions of that period is, perhaps, as much a projection of my own feelings about and memories of Anandapuram when I first visited in the 1980s as it is a reflection of Das's experience. The enormous sense of well-being that had enveloped me during the six months I spent there—my first time away from home, surrounded by people who made me feel welcome, sunshine and palm trees—no doubt shaped the images I now conjured up of Das and his new-found family, cooking Tamil specialities together outside their freshly white-washed mud and thatch house or laughing over a game of carrom board, the images underscored with the scents of jasmine, wood smoke and aromatic spices. And although I knew, intellectually, that the people around me had suffered and were poor—too poor often to buy more than chilli powder to flavour their rice; too poor, sometimes, even to buy rice—I did not experience Anandapuram in that way. Begging took place off-stage, often far away on the other side of the country in Bombay; my stomach was full from meals provided by the kitchen—even if they were sometimes excruciatingly hot; and the warmth and smiles of the people I met often betrayed their hunger and the various domestic crises within which they were embroiled. I was free to enjoy my surroundings in the knowledge that I would be well cared for and could leave at any time. Without a history in the community, I carried no baggage, and could be whatever I wanted to be.[1]

It was not the same for Das: his history was always already there, embodied in his family and in the fact that he, like his father and brother, was a survivor of leprosy. He too was spared begging, though, and not understanding Telugu, at least at first, kept him beyond the unsettling vagaries of village politics and gossip. The family's combined household income also meant they never went hungry, even if he did not, as rumour had it, regularly eat forty idlis in one sitting. "No, no!" he said, rolling his eyes at my gullibility. "It's true that in Brahmin households we might make *prepare* forty or fifty idlis in one batch. My father could very nicely eat twelve, and I could manage six, seven, maybe even eight, because it's our custom to eat them with good *karam pudi*, sambar and chutneys. If we ate like that for breakfast it would keep us full until 1pm. But you couldn't eat forty. The maximum would have to be around twelve. We wouldn't take them two at a time, we'd have the whole lot before us in a big bowl, so maybe that's how it looked to people! And Tamil Brahmins, we'll go more for tiffins than we do for rice, which is what the Andhra people do, so that's another reason why people exaggerate how much we eat!"

Elizabeth Rani or, more often, Timothy, would cook, as, occasionally, would Chandra Prakash. Both men had spent much of their lives before coming to Anandapuram preparing and selling food. They also taught Das's wife, Mariya, later on, although—according to Das—her caste and her background made it hard for her to learn. "Those kinds of people like a lot of hot masalas," he said, implicitly referring to the fact that she was a Madiga. "But our cooking requires subtler spicing: just onions and garlic, turmeric, salt and chilli powder. Non-vegetarian food is cooked in quite a different kind of way." After they moved into their own house in late 1986, where Mariya did all of the cooking, it was years before Das would allow me to eat there: "You don't understand, it won't be suitable for you!" he'd say if I teased him about his failure ever to invite anyone for a meal. "Come to my brother's house instead, and I'll tell him to cook *dahi vada* for you to try instead. He makes the best." The last part at least was true: Chandra Prakash did cook well. But when I did finally sample Mariya's cooking—in the summer of 2007—it all seemed pretty tasty to me.

Das himself never cooked. His days were taken up with work in the office—8am-5pm, six days a week, with, in those early days, a three-hour break in the hottest part of the day, from noon to 3pm. "I'd go back to the house for lunch—rice and curry—sleep for a while, maybe, or read the newspaper and chat to the neighbors, and then go back to the office. Sometimes I'd work late, if there was work to be done, and when I got back I'd bath, eat, sleep. We also had a radio and a tape player, so sometimes we listened to Tamil news and songs. Simple things."

"On Sundays, when there was a bit more time, we'd play cards or dice games just outside by the house, the whole family together. We'd keep a tally of the scores, but we did not play for money—it was just to pass the time.[2] We might say that whoever lost had to make the coffee, or buy some sweets from the teashop. And we'd talk with the neighbors." Rahim, one of the tailors in the colony's weaving unit, and his wife Ameena—Muslims who, like Das, had converted to Christianity—lived next door. "Rahim's wife would tease me a bit, asking me questions in Telugu, and my reply to all her questions was always, 'I'll ask my mother and tell you,' in Telugu, because that was about all I knew how to say! I'd come out with things like, 'I'll come and see you yesterday,' and there was lots of joking and banter about things like that. It helped to pass the time, and for us to get to know one another better."

In the beginning, Das also agreed to attend the local church with his father, although the more he came to understand of the Telugu preachers' messages, the less comfortable he felt with it. It was not, he said, because the message was a Christian rather than a Hindu one. Despite his pride at being a Brahmin, he had, by his own admission, never been a "deep devotee," and Jesus was anyway as worthy of worship as any of the Hindu Gods he knew. "I know already that they are only going to talk about their God, about how he was born, his life, his message, that kind of thing. Hindus tell those kinds of stories about Krishna and the other Gods in the same way. That's all fine. It gives you guidance on how to live your life in a better way. But when I'd been to the temples, you'd not hear Hindu priests blaming others in the same way that you'd hear it in the church. The priests will say that God is great and all that, just as the evangelical fellowship in Anandapuram did, and that was not a problem, but here it wasn't just about celebrating the goodness of God, it was about blaming others as satanic. Sometimes that upset me, that kind of message: they can talk about how great Jesus is, but He never said that we should criticize others. So why do those pastors need to say that if we are worshipping this or that God we will perish? That we will die? If that was true, why are there so many Hindus around doing very nicely, lots of popular, wealthy fellows? They only pray to Hindu Gods, but I don't see them perishing!"

"Perhaps," I said, playing devil's advocate, because I broadly agreed with the point he was making, "they're not talking so much about *now* when they talk about perishing. Perhaps they're referring to the after life, don't you think?"

"It doesn't matter," Das went on, brushing my suggestion aside. "The point is that they do more than just preach a message about God, they talk about how if we do this thing or that thing—if we go to the cinema, for example, or if we smoke cigarettes—then we're going to die, to perish, to burn in hell. What's the value of only cursing us all in that way? God is real, but He's in our hearts, that's what I think, and we need to have faith. But we don't need to go to these prayer meetings where there's lots of weeping and drama, making a big show of it all. People will come along and say that they had a heart problem or something like that, that they saw all these doctors and took all these medicines, but it never got better. And then they go to one prayer meeting, see the light, and get cured in an instant. Now, I can't say whether that's real or not, but I think it's probably a mixture of medicines and faith that has got them better. I may be right, I may be wrong, but that's what I believe. Immediate miracles, maybe we did get them back in ancient times, because back then they didn't know about anything, so whatever happened it seemed like a miracle. But nowadays you can even make babies in test tubes, so where's the need to perform miracles?"

Das paused to take breath, for a moment looking puzzled at where he had ended up. It was unusual for him to talk this passionately about religion. "What was it you were asking?" he said, trying to get back on track. Then: "Ah yes, it was about what we did with our time when I was first here. Well, yes, I did go to church sometimes to start with, but I got fed up with it for the reasons I've talked about, and soon stopped going, except very occasionally, maybe at Easter and those kinds of times."

It was also during his first couple of years in Anandapuram that Das sought a vasectomy reversal operation. He had told neither his wife nor his father that he had even had one in the first place: he had never expected to be in a position to have children, so he had not given it any thought when he got married. Indeed, he claimed he had not even been entirely sure what the operation was for. There were several other men in the village undertaking reversal operations at around the same time, however, which was how he got to know about the possibilities. Men who, like him, had been sterilized during the Emergency made up most of those being operated upon.[3] One of them, a man whose wife was rumoured to be having an affair with a younger man, was said to have wanted the operation so that, if his wife accidentally fell pregnant with her lover's child, he could save face by reasonably claiming that it was his own. Whether the affair was real, a product of village gossip or of the husband's imagination I do not know, but the husband was certainly more open than most in publicizing his operation. I remember it being discussed in the teashop. Das, describing his own decision, did not mention the gossip about the affair, but he did say that it was because of the husband that he had been able to pick up on the details and make his own plans.

He tried to be more discreet about his own operation, telling people he had to have a minor surgery and would need a few days off work. "I went to Dr. Satibabu's private clinic for it and stayed there for a five or six days.

People came to visit me there without knowing what I was in for, although once my father and Elizabeth Rani knew it did not take long for word to get out! Dr. Satibabu told me that I was lucky, that the operation had been very successful, and by experience I now know it was!"

Children were a long way off at that stage, however, and it was work that occupied Das during his first years in the office. The accounts were all hand-written into large ledgers bound with marble-patterned covers, stored away from the termites in an aluminium trunk brightly decorated with painted flowers. Such trunks were common in the days before steel almirahs became ubiquitous, used for storing everything from spices to saris, often stacked high against the back walls of people's one-roomed houses. Moth balls were usually interleaved between the layers of papers or clothes, and the whiff of camphor always transports my mind straight back to Anandapuram. When Solly had done the accounts he had sat, cross-legged, on the floor next to the trunk; Das, like Emma and the typist, Kamala Nehru, who soon joined them, worked at a desk.

"Once I'd discovered the error in the accounting system," he said, "we realized it needed to be done a different way, and so Emma arranged for me to go for some training at another NGO, where they used double-entry book keeping. The English man who ran things there told her I'd need to stay for a month, but after a week, I'd already grasped the system, so I came back early. And it was then I started to realize, I *did* know something, that I could do things. That made me very interested to learn more."

Although staff had their own jobs to do and set office hours, work roles were much less demarcated in the 1980s than they became later on. Someone like Konda Rao, for example, who had worked in both the school and the clinic and eventually managed the elderly people's meals program, was sel-dom where he was expected to be, but he was always willing to pitch in wherever and whenever he was needed. If a foreign visitor needed collecting from the station at 4am, he would invariably be among the welcome party, and he was willing to run errands that had nothing to do with his job descrip-tion. I would bump into him in one or other of the village tea shops, long after the official tea break had ended, helping people to fill in their rail travel concession forms, allowing them a 25 percent discount on fares if they could claim they were travelling for leprosy treatment. "If you ever need ice cream," he once said to me after a tea party he had hosted—and at which he'd served a block of Kwality Neopolitan ice cream—"I'm your man! Just call for me and I can arrange it!" His approach was, perhaps, a throw-back to the *jajmani* relationships people might have been involved in back in their natal villages, where people were tied to one another through a system of caste-based hereditary service relationships.[4] As had once been the case for Das's family back in the village in Thanjavur District, each family would have its own barber, for example, who would be rewarded with an agreed quantity of paddy at harvest time or, perhaps, services in kind. Although these kinds of relationships ceased to exist in Anandapuram—where there were no long-standing ancestral links between families, and where caste no longer operated in the ways it did elsewhere—the notion of work as service, not linked to specific, immediate financial reward, still lingered. Konda Rao, say, would bring me ice cream when required or visit me if I was sick; I, as his patron, might then be called upon to reciprocate when the need arose—when, for example, a medical operation or a marriage feast needed to be funded. Years later, when an outside project co-ordinator was appointed, junior staff members would volunteer to weed his garden or carry out minor repairs in his house. They did not expect these tasks to be directly remunerated, but they did expect, in a non-specified kind of way, protection and favour in return. It was a set of arrangements that took me a very long time to understand.

Das, perhaps because he was a Brahmin, perhaps because he had grown-up in towns and cities, away from extended kinship networks, did not treat anyone quite as a patron. Nevertheless, his attitude to work was shaped by the same service attitude rather than by a calculation of how much money he would be paid per hour. It also, from his perspective, made work much more interesting, and he was quite happy to stack his ledgers back in the trunk box and take off to buy a box of zips—very difficult to get hold of on the open market in Andhra Pradesh back then—via contacts back in Madras. "I knew Tamil and Hindi as well as English," Das reminded me, "so if work needed doing in another state it was easy to send me to deal with it." There was a federation of producer associations through which Anandapuram had begun to export its woven products called Tradefair, and its main offices were in Madras. "Because I could understand Tamil, if Emma was too busy with other work to attend meetings and workshops down there, she started to send me. This was in about 1987, a couple of years after I left the station, and I liked the way they treated me there. Dignity and respect were new things to me, I never expected to have them, but when I went to those offices to attend meetings, the employees there would treat me like a sir! I even started to help them with organizing exhibitions and other things."

"I didn't spend much time with the people I'd known on the station when I went back through Madras," he went on, "I'd just greet them and tell them that I had this job in Andhra. They'd be pleased for me—their attitude would be that one of our people had found a proper job, had managed to get off the station, so they'd be proud. Back then, I'd spent my time mixing with mostly poor, low-caste people, and running from the police and other authorities. Now I was starting to move with officials and educated people, even foreigners. And I came to realize that it wasn't all about high educational qualifications and background, that it was possible to be accepted in higher circles without all those things. I'd go wherever I was sent, and I'd do my best in

English, I wouldn't worry if I got the grammar right or not, but I'd make myself understood, and it was only then—when I started mixing with these people—that I realized even people with degrees and other qualifications were often more afraid about speaking English than I had been! So I started to appreciate what my experiences had given me."

Das continued: "Foreigners would come—like this electrician from England—and I'd go to meet them, travel with them and learn from them. When I met the electrician and his wife they wanted to travel first class, so I went first class with them too, and they even took me with them for food at a five-star hotel!"

The biggest boost to Das's growing confidence, though, came when he stood in for Emma on a micro-entrepreneurship training course. "They sent her an invitation, and she couldn't go, but she replied asking if she could send a representative. The real cost of the training was quite high, but because we were coming from a leprosy colony, she asked if they could subsidize us, and they agreed. This was my first proper training, and there were big people, officers and the like, there. I arrived on the first evening—it was residential—and they opened with a party: sodas, alcoholic drinks and everything on offer. I was only in ordinary working clothes—shirt and trousers—and I was afraid at first. 'How can I manage with all these high up people?' I thought! I didn't even take alcohol then, so I just had a *Thums Up!* cola and found a couple of other Tamil speakers to talk with."

The big change in how he saw himself and those around him came the next morning: "I remember, the class sessions began, and the man who organized the whole thing was talking us through these calculations. I sat quietly for a while, not wanting to answer any of his questions. I was aware I was uneducated and didn't want to look foolish in front of all these people. Most of the other participants, I think, had just come to spend money, to have a change of scene and to enjoy the food and the drink. They were used to this kind of workshop. But I was concentrating on the calculations, and, after a while, I started to put my hand-up to give the answer. 'That was quick,' the teacher said, surprised at how fast I'd come up with the solution. 'Do you have a calculator there?' I told him that I hadn't, that I'd just worked out the answer myself. He was impressed, although I didn't really notice it at the time because I was busy concentrating. It was only later that I realized I *did* know things, even if I hadn't had all this formal education. And after I came back from that course the organizer sent Emma a letter of praise, saying how well I had learned."

The letter meant a lot to Das, and still does. He has a yellowing copy of it in the flimsy file of important documents he keeps on a shelf in the corner of his house, along with a couple of photographs of his family from the local photo studio and his school leaving certificate. In the letter, the course organizer notes that Das "has a mind like a computer" and that he had been wrong to think he was not up to the course. "He has low self-confidence," reads the letter, "but he shouldn't have—this man is a real gem." Like the meetings with his brother and his father on the station, this training course and its consequences makes it into most renderings of Das's life story: another pivotal event in his life history. He had begun to think himself worthy of the job of Financial Controller, which is what his job title became in 1987 after another foreigner, a woman from England called Wanda who came to help re-establish Anandapuram's rehabilitation programs as potentially profit-making businesses, suggested his promotion. Wanda had spent time with Das costing and pricing the goods that were being made in the weaving unit, and was impressed at how much he knew. "He had *all* the details stored there in his head," Emma told me when I asked her about it later. "He had a real way with figures: it was something that stood out to people."

After Wanda left, she donated her Amstrad computer and a mountain of large floppy disks, all of which arrived via sea mail a few months later. Das had already learned the rudiments of using a keyboard back at the typing institute in Madras after he left school; the rest—he told me—he was able to pick up by following the onscreen step-by-step instructions. "I started doing occasional letter typing and other things," he said, "and began using the computer to produce spreadsheets and other materials we needed for the accounts. I was very slow at first, but I put a lot of time into learning, and gradually my skills improved."

By now, the office had also moved out of the circular mud and thatch hut where it had been accommodated for the past few years and into a larger, purpose built brick and cement building that also housed the weaving and sewing unit. Funded by a UK charitable trust, the new office also sported electric ceiling fans and proper shelving for Das's ledgers and other files, and it looked—for the first time—like a professional office. Whether this professionalisation was good, bad or something inbetween is a matter of opinion, but one positive upshot of capital investment in Anandapuram, according to Das, was "there was plenty of money around in the accounts that enabled us to pay salaries on time and the rice bills. We had good cash flow." Too much cash flow, as will become apparent later, also opened the door to a whole other set of problems, but for the time being it made relations between the administration and the 200 or so staff working in Anandapuram's programs—from the weaving unit to the school and the clinic—much more plain sailing.

It was also in 1987 that Das's father, Timothy, set about arranging his younger son's marriage. It was a much grander affair than Das and Mariya's had been. "They spent lakhs of rupees!" Das told me. "Chandra Prakash had been begging with my father and step-mother for a few years by then, so they had more money around than when I got married, and anyway, I hadn't been interested in a big meeting." A match was found from another leprosy colony that Anandapuram had links with in Vizags, and preparations were put in place. There was a wedding feast for the entire colony, and even two of Gajavakra's brothers from Tamil Nadu attended.

Things went well at first for Chandra Prakash and his new wife, Rani, even though no children were forthcoming. Chandra Prakash had not had a vasectomy like Das, but he had, he told me candidly, a low sperm count, possibly caused either by his leprosy or his treatment for it. The same local doctor who had undertaken Das's vasectomy reversal operation also treated him though, so he was hopeful that conception was just a matter of time. However, according both to Chandra Prakash and Das, the women Rani befriended in the Colony were a bad influence on her. On June 15, 1990—Chandra Prakash remembered the precise date—she did what, until that point, had been the preserve of men in Das's family: she absconded along with two other women. Chandra Prakash kept his story at that. In his version, she absconded, finally came back, and then he divorced her. Das, who I felt more comfortable to push for further information, volunteered more detail: "Everyone suspected that two brothers were involved," said Das, naming the notorious sons of one of the village Elders. "One of them was sleeping with one of the girls who absconded, that's what everyone thought, so when they returned—a month or two later—the girls were called to the storeroom to give their accounts of what had happened."

The storeroom—so called because it was used to house government rations of rice and other basic provisions to be distributed, at set low-rates, to ration card holders in Anandapuram—was also the community hall, and the place where justice was metered out by the Elders. Any member of the colony could pay a small fee to "ring the bell" which hung in front of the storeroom. The sound summonsed not just the accused parties and the Elders, who were responsible for making judgement, but anyone in the colony who was interested to hear the case. In the early days, back in the 1960s, those suspected of adultery were sometimes tied up there and physically beaten; by the 1980s, punishments were less likely to be corporal. The guilty tended to be fined or banished from the village for a while.

"But when the girls came back, they were not telling the truth about why they left or where they had been," Das told me. "Maybe they were afraid because they had had connections with other men while they were gone. But at that time, if Rani had told the truth and said sorry, then my family would have been prepared to take her back. Rani continued to tell lies though. In front of everyone she said that Chandra Prakash was not able to perform sex, that he was impotent. I don't think she knew what she was saying: she'd been coached to say this by the other girls. They'd told her she wouldn't be punished so harshly if she said something like that. We couldn't accept this. Her words hurt our family, so we couldn't agree to take her back to our home. Still the Elders and others tried to convince her, in the store, to admit that she was telling lies, that she had been coached to say those things about her husband. But we said no, even if she apologizes now, it's too late. We said that she would have to go back to her mother and father."

"They claimed they were Reddys, those people—high caste, in this area—but they turned out to be worse than Malas and Madigas!" Das proclaimed bitterly. These unpleasant events marked, in his mind, the beginning of his family's change in fortunes. "Until around that time, we were very popular in the colony," he recalled. "I'd started to learn Telugu by then so did lots of the translations at meetings between the Elders and Emma or at public events, so I was a well-known face. And Elizabeth Rani, although she sometimes gave Mariya a difficult time, she wasn't like she became a few years later. We were respected."

It was in 1990, the same year that Chandra Prakash's wife absconded, that Elizabeth Rani, in Das's words, "became half mental." The initial catalyst was Timothy's decision—without discussing it with his wife—to sell the brick-built house they had been allotted as part of a major house building scheme in the colony, and to invest the proceeds, and more besides, in rebuilding the house on their current plot. Her objections, it seems, were many and varied, but the main one, other than his decision to act unilaterally, was that he had sold at too low a price and had paid too much for the upgrading of their existing place, putting them in debt. Das offered no comment on whether he thought she was justified in her anger, although Timothy's previous record on managing his finances suggests that she might well have had a point. Judging by the gold ornaments Elizabeth Rani liked to adorn herself with, though, it is probably also fair to say that Timothy's second wife's tastes were more expensive to accommodate than those of his first.

"Up until then she wasn't too bad," Das told me. "There had been small fights between her and Mariya, my wife, but mostly we managed to put a stop to those quite quickly. Elizabeth Rani would bemoan the fact that she'd given her family money and that she'd brought nothing herself, and Mariya would get upset, shout and then weep. But my brother and my father, they wouldn't leave her to cry, and Chandra Prakash would tell Elizabeth Rani to leave her alone. And then, in 1987, when the new houses were built, we got one of our own, so Mariya and I moved there, and it became easier."

Now, however, Elizabeth Rani's fury at Timothy was spilling out into everything. "Even though he was working hard and begging and cooking," Das said, "she'd make more and more demands. She kept on at him, all of the time. She became cruel. She'd yell at him, 'you did this, you did that, you are not giving a single paise to me, you sold my house, you don't want to do anything for me,' that kind of thing, all of the time." Chandra Prakash, already suffering at the humiliating breakdown of his marriage, found the situation almost unbearable. "He'd cry out at her, 'Why do you shout at my father like this!,' and he got so upset he started hitting himself on the head with the tea-making vessel. It was a good, German-made aluminium one, and he hit himself so hard it broke! That's how upset he was!"

At the time Das was telling me this—sitting on the verandah of the guest house drinking sweet tea, the fan cutting lazily through the humid air—the idea of hitting oneself over the head with a metal teapot in protest at events spiralling out of control did not seem an unreasonable one. Self-harm was, after all, a fairly common response to circumstances one felt otherwise powerless to intervene in, and were, as in the case of Mariya's step-father's overdose of leprosy drugs, often remarkably successful in bringing about a desired change. My field notes were littered with tales of fathers gorging themselves on hot green chillies in near deadly quantities to get their daughters to do what they wanted, or of daughters quaffing litre bodies of phenyl in protest at being prevented from marrying their paramours. When such actions did not kill those who undertook them, they invariably got their own way.[5]

Luckily, Chandra Prakash's own frustrations were short lived, and his luck was about to improve. Israel, one of the Elders and also a pastor in Anandapuram, had heard through a fellow pastor, who lived in the Vizags leprosy colony, about a girl in his care. Like Chandra Prakash, she was a young divorcee, and, on hearing about what had happened with Rani, was keen to put herself forward as a potential marriage partner. "She was from the same colony as Rani," said Das, "and she'd heard good things about him. I think her own first husband had beaten her, and she knew Chandra Prakash wasn't like that. She also knew that it was going to be harder to find someone for a girl who had already been married, so Chandra Prakash seemed like the answer to her prayers."

Chandra Prakash had, after his earlier experience, been understandably reticent in the face of his father's cajoling him to remarry, but since this girl had come forward herself to express interest, he was prepared to consider it. They eventually married in April 1991. "And even that wasn't a small affair!" Das recalled. "If they spent Rs40,000 on the first one, they must have spent about Rs25,000 on this one. But it was important to make a show of it after what had happened with Rani. We needed to show that what she was saying about him was all lies."

Chandra Prakash stopped begging after his first marriage. When building of the new houses began in 1986—a massive project funded by the Indian government and overseas charities—sand was excavated from the ground to be mixed with the cement. The resulting hole was turned into a fish tank, and Chandra Prakash was given the task, for daily wages, of maintaining it. He proved himself a hard worker, moving on from that to gardening work, later into the new plastics moulding unit and, much later still, into the central kitchen, where he helped prepare meals for the elderly. He also acquired a cycle rickshaw, which he pulled privately after working hours were over. His new wife, Sara, worked part-time in the weaving unit and, although their joint income was hardly substantial—and less than it would have been when he was begging—they managed to get by.

Das's own marriage lacked the drama of Chandra Prakash's first, and maybe that made Das appreciate Mariya more than he might otherwise have done, but he was never enthusiastic about the match. Even back in 1986, when they had been married less than a year, Das was already expressing resignation: it was not her fault, he always maintained, but they were not suitable for one another. Although he found a great satisfaction in his work and the newfound appreciation of his skills, his ascendance made the contrast between his professional position—as a respected man in the village and beyond, with skills at managing the accounts—and the lack of satisfaction in his marriage to a low-caste woman with whom he could scarcely converse even more pronounced.

"At the time I'd gone along with it partly because I didn't think there would be another chance to find someone at my age," he lamented, "but Kamala Nehru, the typist in the office, she was very interested in me. If I'd waited another year, things could have been very different." Kamala Nehru had arrived in 1986, a recruit from the neighbouring town. Das was not sure what her caste was—she was a converted Christian, so probably not a very high one—but she was educated and could speak some English. In Das's imagination, she would have served the role of wife much better than his own: she knew, in his terms, "how to move in the world." Kamala Nehru was older than Mariya, pleasantly plump and plainly, but neatly, dressed. Mariya, by contrast, always had a look of wildness about her in Das's eyes: her thick curly hair, although tied back, always looked as though it was struggling to escape, and ever deeper frown lines were already beginning to form above her heavy brows. Although she was, according to Das, devoted to him, she was shy and, I think, lonely in Anandapuram. Although there were some exchanges with the other women in their street—they shared a couple of grinding stones and often ground spices, or the dhals for *idli*s, communally—Das said that she never formed any real friendships with any of them. "She was quick to take offense at things other women said, or she'd think I was siding with them against her, but if she and another woman are yelling at each other in the street, I have to tell her to stop and come inside, no? She's my wife, so she's the one I have to command. But she takes that to mean I am taking the other woman's side against her. That's how she thinks."

The physical side of their relationship was also difficult, probably aggravated by Mariya's persistent anemia and other minor ailments, mostly consequences of the poverty of her short childhood. When no children appeared in the first years after Das's vasectomy reversal operation he was not surprised: "She was not very willing, I always had to work hard to convince her, and we probably had sexual relations only about fifteen or twenty times in those first eight years," he said. "But finally, one day she complained about some chest pain, and we noticed there was some swelling in her stomach. Sara took her to the hospital, and the doctor confirmed that she had conceived. I was pleased, and I tried to take good care of her, to make sure she ate good things. And she was very happy."

Mariya remained anemic, however, and the slightness of her frame also mitigated against a straightforward delivery. When the time came, Das said, she needed a caesarean, and she was admitted to Dr. Satibabu's nursing home. "At 1:30am in the morning on March 15, 1995, the baby was finally born. It was a boy. Half of the people from our street were there in the hospital, and it was a happy time, a time of great celebration for our family. Mariya's family was pleased too. He was strong and healthy and, a year later, the pastor gave him the name Joshua."

Not only had they been blessed with a son, Das told me, but their son brought them good luck. Timothy, at the time of Joshua's birth, had been critically ill. "He had fallen sick while begging with Elizabeth Rani in Bombay, and I had to go to Tirupathi to collect him and bring him to the hospital," Das remembered. "We thought at that time he would die. The doctor said there was no hope. But as my father always said, his grandson was on the way then, and that changed the course of his life, that's why he recovered. We took care of him, and he survived."

So despite a souring of relations with Elizabeth Rani, the absconding of Chandra Prakash's first wife and the disappointment of his own marriage, Das was mostly positive about his life into the earlier half of the 1990s. He spoke better Telugu now, and this had enabled better communication with other men in the village. He now played badminton and other games with them outside the storeroom in the early evenings after work. There were weekend family bicycle and rickshaw trips to the beach, around six miles away, to watch the sun rise or set and eat chapattis, potatoes flavoured with chillies and cumin and yellow with turmeric, and chutney made from the local spinach-like green leaf, *gongora*. Women would paddle, fully dressed in their saris, while men and children would strip down to their underpants and leap through the waves, often, in the case of the men, fortified by a nip or two of cheap whisky to "give them bravery." Groups of men, Das among them, also went on occasional longer cycle rallies, including one I took part in early in 1987 to Nagarjuna Sagar Dam, one hundred-miles inland. The atmosphere on such trips was carefree—young men cut free from the responsibilities of work and family—and Das was in high spirits, bantering with the others in ways that his work in the office did not always allow him to.

By mid-1995, however, other changes in the village were also afoot.

NOTES

1. I am reminded again here of Alter, *Knowing Dil Das*, and the outwardly obscured differences between First World anthropologists and their global south interlocutors that his account of Dil Das's friendships brings out so starkly.

2. Jeffrey, *Timepass* (a & b).

3. For more on the Government's family planning programs, see Carolyn Henning Brown, "The Forced Sterilization Program Under the Indian Emergency: Results in One Settlement," *Human Organization*, 43, 1 (1984): 49–54; A. Dharmalingam, "The Social Context of Family Planning In a South Indian Village," *International Family Planning Perspectives*, 21, 3 (1995): 98–103; Tarlo, *Unsettling Memories*; Toofan, *When Freedom Bleeds*.

4. Mayer, "Inventing village tradition"; C. J. Fuller, "Misconceiving the grain heap."

5. Staples, "The suicide niche"; Staples, "Ethnographies of Suicide in South Asia"; Staples and Widger, "Situating Suicide as an Anthropological Problem."

Chapter Seven

The Rise . . .

There had always been a tension in Anandapuram between projects that are externally funded and run by the central administration, on the one hand, and areas managed by the elected village elders—who were entirely responsible for community affairs, from the arrangement of marriages to administering local justice—on the other. Whereas other colonies were run from above, with the "inmates," as they were sometimes referred to, told what to do by the NGOs that ran them, Anandapuram had never been like that. Self-started and self-run, outside help had come in at a later point in its history, and the form which that help took was always subject to the Elders' approval.

This arrangement did not always make lines of authority in Anandapuram's projects very clear, but it was also one of the things that had attracted volunteers like Emma Cox to work there. Whatever the messy realities of actually getting things done, her aim was not to make up the rules herself and offer them on a take-it-or-leave-it basis, but to work with the people of Anandapuram to attain the services they needed and, from their perspective, deserved. Compared to what seemed like the stifling environments of some colonies, where residents were given very specific tasks to perform in exchange for rations of food, medical care and perhaps a small financial allowance, the approach taken in Anandapuram, especially to a western outsider like me, seemed refreshingly progressive.

So while Emma ran the office as administrator, it was, at least technically, the Elders who were calling the shots. It was their village, and the office existed to serve it. When there were appointments to be made, the Elders expected to have a say in who would be given the jobs, and they also wanted a say in how the funds that came in to the village were spent. This was not an easy situation to work with, particularly as the projects and the amounts of money that were coming in to the community got bigger. Donors funded particular projects and wanted to see returns on their investments, or at least evidence that the money had been spent as they intended it. Donations also came with caveats: demands that women were equally represented in the decision making process, for example, or that grants promoted self-reliance.[1] The Elders, all male, tended to see women, foreign women excepted, as unsuitable for decision-making. They were, moaned an Elder at one meeting I attended, too prone to gossip to be fully trusted. Staff, whether from inside the community or outside, also expected some form of job security and to have their salaries paid regularly and on time, whether the Elders considered that a priority or not. The Elders' right to remove a person from a colony job and replace him or her with someone else, however, was a significant aspect of their political power. It enabled them to punish those who appeared to work against them, and to reward those who were on their side.

Another issue was that although elections of Elders were supposed to take place only once a year, in reality they occurred far more often. Plotting by adversaries or accusations that they had "eaten the money" often led to them being over-turned in monthly general body meetings, when all male members of the colony congregated together, and for new sets of Elders to be put in their place. While the Elders tended to be made up of seven of the same twenty or so people constantly jostling for power, the instability of their positions could, one might argue, mitigate against good, longer term decision making in favour of quick fix political strategies that would buy them electoral support. Not so different, on reflection, from most democratically elected governments the world over.

Emma and her colleagues in the office—Das among them—debated and struggled with the Elders over routine affairs on an almost daily basis. Until a separate meeting room was established specifically to house those meetings, they would regularly bring work in the main office to a halt, when the seven of them would troop in and sit down in a circle on the floor with Emma and Das, who helped with translation as well as putting his own point of view across. The Elders were all male and, although not necessarily old, were mostly drawn from the earlier settlers. Consequently, they displayed the most classic forms of leprosy impairments. Many of them had lost fingers and toes through muscle wastage and operations, or their noses had collapsed, creating the leonine features associated with the disease. They would arrive with a clatter of crutches on the concrete floor of the office, all the better to wave expressively above their heads if the need arose. A pile of leprosy-footwear outside the entrance was a sign that they were inside. Although they described themselves as "patients," however, there was never anything passive about the group, and it was, perhaps, this resilience and furious energy that made them compelling as well as sometimes difficult to work with.

They had, after all, established this community themselves, despite not only having a stigmatized disease and, in some cases, major physical impairments. They had also been penniless, uneducated and institutionalized. The more I thought about it, the more inspiring their achievements seemed. Nevertheless, their unannounced arrivals at the office certainly had a discernible impact on the level of work that went on inside. The Elders were seldom well-briefed on the precise financial situation or on how funds had already been earmarked and they were often frustrated at their incapacity to get money spent on the new projects they wanted to promote. The latter were more likely to be hand-out type programs of the kind that donors, by then, were less keen to fund: they wanted to see evidence, at least on paper, of development. On the ground, if the President or Secretary had been gifted money by a family who wanted a precious colony job for, say, their son, there would also be a strong push by the Elders to get that boy in post, regardless of his qualifications for whatever job might be available.

If the Elders were difficult to manage at times, the general colony population often seemed even worse. Expectations and aspirations were high and, because of the money that did come in—often rather less than was imagined on the streets—there was competition to get a slice of it, either in the form of a job or welfare benefits, that simply did not exist in the same way in other villages. This meant that when the Elders were not traipsing in and out of the office, individuals often were, whether to complain about the medicines they had been prescribed by the clinic—by paramedics who were sometimes accused of trying to poison their patients, or at the very least trying to fob them off with less expensive and less effective drugs—or the quality and quantity of food being served by the kitchen.

I worked in the office as a volunteer for a second time between August 1986 and February 1987, and was often left speechless at the kind of enquiries that came in to the office or, out of hours, to wherever you happened to be. Someone woke me early one Sunday morning by hammering on my door, only to present me with an aluminium pot half-full of chicken curry. "That looks nice," I said, bleary eyed. The man who had given it to me, a recipient of the Colony's meals program, snatched it back. "But look at the size of the portion they've given me!" he said, outraged, before demanding that I somehow right the situation. I felt cornered and helpless, but at least, as an outsider, I had an escape. For senior office staff like Das who lived in the Colony, the continuous demands were relentless and wearing.

On another day an elderly man came in to the office to complain that one of the arms of his spectacles had come loose, and wanted to know what we were going to do about it. It was towards the end of a long day, and we stared back at him, jaws dropped open in disbelief. Enquiries like that, in temperatures that sometimes went beyond 45 degrees Celsius and when the electricity supply was off—as it often was in those days of load shedding, as the electricity company called it—induced a kind of inertia. But they also produced a certain camaraderie among the staff and a corresponding dark humour, at which Das was a master.

Sometimes though, complainants went further, as was the case a few months prior to my visit in 1995. The father of a newly still-born baby, wracked with grief, came wailing into the office to blame the staff for their lack of support in getting his wife to the hospital for her delivery sooner. Holding the baby, wrapped in swaddling, he marched through the office and threw the dead body down in front of Emma and Das on the desk. "How can you keep your sanity when this sort of thing is going on all the time?" asked Das, rhetorically, as he recalled the incident. The memory still made him shudder. "We need at least to be polite about how we do things, no? This was an office, for God's sake!"

It was also in 1995 that things came to a head between Emma and the Elders. Earlier in the year, the Elders had removed three young men from their Colony jobs; all the healthy sons of parents affected by leprosy. As they were not members of the association, however, none of them could attend or vote at general body meetings, so could neither become Elders nor affect the outcome of elections. It was against this background that the three dismissed men had become founding members of the Youth Welfare Society (YWS), a separate association—complementary or oppositional to the Elders, depending on one's perspective—focused on finding support for the healthy but, as they saw it, stigmatized sons of people with leprosy. The Society drew heavily on support from the local Telugu Desam Party (TDP), which had been in power in the State since the 1994 assembly elections. Although the TDP's leader was then the popular film star N T Rama Rao—the god-like character Das's boss in Madras had been a neighbour to in the late 1960s—Colony members had always voted for the opposing Congress Party. It had been local Congress councillors, Elders told me, who had helped them when they first established the colony, and, although it was custom to accept gifts and alcoholic drinks from *all* the parties at election times, the Elders had always directed the villagers to vote for the Congress. The YWS's dalliance with the TDP was seen as a direct threat to this state of affairs; the removal of three of the Society's leaders from their jobs was a show of authority by the older generation. [2]

In the past, those who felt they had been hard done by would have rung the bell in the storeroom and the matter would have been settled internally. Even when a colony man had punched another during a drunken brawl, and his adversary, hitting his head on the concrete path beneath him had died, no-one had considered it necessary to involve the police or the law courts. The Elders had considered the case and, accepting that it had been an accident, had ordered the survivor of the fight to give financial support to the widow and family of the deceased. The younger generation, however, was not so ready to accept the authority of a group of Elders they had had no role in electing, and they backed the three men who had been sacked in taking their case to an outside industrial tribunal. A letter had arrived from their lawyers at around the time I arrived in the village for a three-week holiday in the summer of 1995, citing Emma and Das, by then her unofficial deputy, as their employers.[3]

By the time I left the village, the rift between those on the side of the dismissed workers—who were increasingly angry—and the Elders was becoming increasingly entrenched, and Emma was having little success in getting the situation resolved to her satisfaction. When an unexpected offer of a job for another NGO that worked with people affected by leprosy based in Bangalore came out of the blue in late August, Emma decided to take it. She had spent nearly fifteen years in Anandapuram, but it felt like the right time to move on. Within a month, she had gone. Her resignation at least provided the jolt the Elders needed to reinstate those they had sacked, and the YWS also ceased its operations for a while. A period of relative calm ensued, one that the Elders initially thought would be sufficient to provoke a withdrawal of Emma's resignation, but she had made up her mind.

It was this state of affairs that led to Das being catapulted into the number one position in Anandapuram: the newly created role of Administrative Officer. It was also the background to this situation that set the scene for his term in office and for many of the difficulties he faced. A lot of people in the village were shaken or numb at the departure of "their ammagaru." There had also been a long-established belief that the community's programs could never be managed by anyone other than a foreigner, and certainly not by one of their own members. Das had a lot to live up to. As one of the men had said during a meeting before I left Anandapuram: "We need to have foreigners here to run things. Indians don't think about doing service, they won't look after us properly."

At this stage, however, Das was still generally respected and well-liked within the village, and he had the support of a newly-formed management committee—a group comprising representatives of the Elders, outside donors, and locals of high standing that was tabled to meet three or four times a year to rule on policy—so he claimed not to have been too daunted by the prospect of the role. "I didn't want it, especially," he said, with a shrug of his shoulders, "and I wasn't convinced I was able to do it, but it felt like a duty, and I tried to follow what Emma had done when she was in the post. If there wasn't money available to buy rice for the old people's meals program we'd take loans in the bazaar, get rice on credit. That was how it had always been done. When Jack left, there were outstanding bills of Rs1.5 lakhs that Emma dealt with; by the time she left, we owed more than double that to the shops, and I had to manage the repayments."

He was also acutely aware of additional problems: "There was an extra burden because funds for the clinic were decreasing. Leprosy was seen as being on the way out and there wasn't the money around for it that there had been in the past. And as the weaving unit got bigger, so did the subsidies we needed to support it. Then there was special medical care: we had more and more patients who were living longer but who got other conditions that we needed to look after. Before, these people would just have died earlier on. Now they lived and had heart attacks and other things that we needed to treat them for. But we continued to provide everything, to balance one thing off against another. We did fall behind with provident fund (PF) payments for staff, though, because there wasn't enough always in the pot to pay both salaries and PF, so we'd think we'd deal with that later. One month we'd get some money in and pay off the rice bill, another month some more would come in and we'd use it for something else. That's how we worked."

On paper, Das's role looked relatively straightforward, even if his duties were far-reaching. Each of the departments, from the clinic to the school, had their own heads, and Das's job was to manage them on a day-to-day basis; to ensure statutory paperwork was submitted to the relevant authorities; and to oversee spending. He was also responsible for communicating with donors—producing a newsletter and annual reports—and for ensuring outside visitors were well looked after. A typical day, if there was such a thing, might include a visit to the weaving unit to check on the progress of an order; a lively meeting with the Elders; and some letter writing and form-filling. But as the tensions I have already described suggest, the job turned out to be more stressful than a simple list of Das's duties implies, and this was only partly because of the demands of the job itself.

A major issue was Das's management of his own money. Although he always talks about his personal debts coming later, I know for certain—because of concerns that Emma had shared with me when we met that summer—that he owed moneylenders around Rs 42,000 in 1995. He had confided in Emma about this some months earlier, as the two of them returned from a business trip to Chennai. They were travelling on a cycle rickshaw from the railway station to the colony in the dead of night when the story came out. Sitting side-by-side on a rickshaw, which allowed intimacy without eye contact, and under the cover of darkness was often Das's preferred context for making revelations (an insight which served me well in finding out the details of his story). He was anxious and losing sleep, he told her, because his debts had grown so big. The amount seems rather small now, particularly given the size his dues swelled to later on. However, for a man who, until his promotion to Administrative Officer, had been earning around Rs3,000 per month, it was a significant sum. Moneylenders within Anandapuram usually charged between 3 and 5 percent interest per month, while outside lenders charged as much as 10 percent. Das's interest payments alone were likely to have been over Rs2,000—the lion's share of his salary—leaving him next to nothing to live on and a debt that was never getting any smaller. Even after his salary increase, which took him up to about Rs5,000 per month, he was struggling: there were also chit funds, long since drawn, that he was committed to paying into, and a proportion of his salary was also cut at source every month to pay back advances and other debts to the office.

Das also told me that it was not until after Emma had left and that his circumstances in the village became increasingly difficult that he turned again to gambling on cards and horse racing and took up drinking. His debts, he said, had started small with loans to help cover the cost of family events, such as his brother's weddings or the spiralling costs of renovation works on his father's house. They had increased to the levels they were at in 1995 through growing interest repayments. Family expenditure had remained constant, so, when one lender demanded money, he had borrowed from another to pay missing instalments to the first. He insists they were nothing to do with what he referred to as "habits."

"Mariya, my wife," he said, "was never good with money. If the flower seller came along and told her it was Rs5 for a measure of jasmine, that's what she'd give him, no haggling or anything. The real price should have been about Rs2."

"But surely," I responded cynically, "you didn't ratchet up your debts by Mariya overpaying for jasmine? That would take an awful lot of flowers . . ."

"Ah, it builds up!"he replied, testily. "But it wasn't just flowers. If a man selling aluminium pans came to the door to sell her one—or anyone came selling anything—she'd just buy it, no questions, no arguing over the price, nothing. There was no control over spending."

Given that Mariya had limited access to cash and seldom strayed far from the house, other than to her part-time job in the weaving unit, I was unconvinced that she was the source of his debts. We often argued about it over the years to come. Unlike Elizabeth Rani, Mariya wore no gold ornaments—just a couple of glass bangles, if anything—and her saris were not expensive, even if she did buy them very occasionally from passing hawkers. The theory of increasing interest charges on unpaid debts seemed the more plausible of his explanations at the time, but even this did not convince me entirely.

It was not just the fact that Das had no money that was the problem, however, but who he owed it to. Wesley, the accounts clerk who had worked under Das when he was Financial Controller and had taken on the title of Accounts Officer when Das was promoted, was also one of the village's most successful moneylenders, and it was to him he owed a large chunk of his debt. Wesley's money had come, people in the village claimed, from his mother-in-law. He had invested it cannily—mainly in those in the village who needed quick cash, and who then repaid at interest rates of three per cent per month. Although Wesley's rates were generous compared to those of outside lenders, many of his debtors could still not afford to repay the capital.

This suited Wesley well, as it did other moneylenders, because it ensured an almost continuous income.

In Das's case, it also weakened his position as Wesley's boss. If Wesley demanded overtime payments in order to complete the accounts work, it was difficult for Das to deny him. And although Das claims that Wesley never received any special treatment because of their financial ties outside the office, most of Das's other lenders were also staff members under his command, and I was concerned that this made him vulnerable.

With retrospect, I wonder if we exaggerated the potential risk that Emma's departure had on donors' willingness to give to Anandapuram. We may have given too much credence to the villagers' own beliefs that only foreigners were capable of looking after them properly, while most donors were more concerned with whether there were structures in place to receive their donations rather than who would be administering them. At the time though, it was a very real fear, and both Emma and Anandapuram's charity in England were keen to ensure that Das had all the support he needed. Back in the UK, I had been working for five years as a journalist on a trade magazine, and I was becoming restless. Another six-month trip to India, it seemed, could be the solution both to my itchy feet and to Das's need of some visible support. I gave in my notice and planned to return to the village in March 1996.

Meanwhile, I also discussed Das's debt problem with the charity's committee. I talked to Das about it too, although it was difficult: these were the days before email and cheap telephone connections. If I had a question to ask him I had to send a letter and wait another two or three weeks for the reply. If he had misunderstood the question, or had chosen not to answer it, I would either have to write again or give up. Nevertheless, with the help of the charity's chairman, Marcus, we were able to make a plan. Marcus agreed to lend Das the £800 he needed to pay off his debts, which he would repay in manageable instalments every month into a building society account. Das would send us a photocopy of the account's passbook every month to demonstrate that he was paying the money back. When Marcus came to India, as he planned to do in a few years' time, he would collect the money. There would be no interest payments, so the debt would genuinely decrease every month.

I was thrilled that we had found a solution. I was to take the money with me in travellers' checks, change it into rupees in a bank in Madras, and then take the money back to Das. He was to repay it to his creditors directly, so that they would not be alerted to the fact that we had lent him the money. The committee, I recall, was concerned that, if word got out, others in the village might justifiably have been irked that he was receiving special treatment when they all had debts of their own. Again, with retrospect, transparency might have worked better, but, at the time, I rather enjoyed the intrigue and

the thrill of travelling back from Madras with my small, nondescript back-
pack stuffed full of crisp banknotes. Thankfully, I was not robbed.

Das though apparently had been, which is why he was having to repay a
debt to the office. When Emma was still there, late in 1994 or early in 1995,
he had made one of his visits to Madras to buy zips for the weaving unit on
the black market. Before he got them he was, he claimed, pick pocketed,
losing all the Rs19,000 he had on him. It was something that happened to
him twice more over the next decade. He may have been unlucky or, if he
had been drinking, careless. It might also have been because he was in places
where he was not supposed to have been—like the race course—and had not
been paying proper attention to the money in his pocket. He always denied
losing the money on the horses though, an activity which, he claimed consis-
tently, never left him with a significant loss.

Trips to the races, Das told me, had only re-started in around 1990, when
the family's problems that resulted in Chandra Prakash hitting himself with
the German teapot were just beginning. A couple of times in our conversations he seemed to date it earlier, but it certainly preceded playing cards for
money with other colony men. "Between 1985 and 2005 I never played cards
here," he said. "I was working in the office and then became the project co-
ordinator, so it would have been disrespectful to sit on the roadside and play
openly. But if I got the chance to go out—which wasn't very often—sometimes I'd go and place a few small bets on the horses. Only a couple of times
though, not much."

A trip to the race course in Madras, Das claimed, was any way better
value than going to the cinema back at home. "If I'd been sent to Madras for
some business, I'd try to find time to go the races. It would cost between
Rs10 and Rs30—maybe Rs50 if you went for the air conditioned accommodation—and you could go there at 9 o'clock in the morning and stay there
until 6 o'clock in the evening, a whole day's entertainment. In Andhra Pradesh it was illegal, but it wasn't in Madras, nor in other foreign countries,
like the United Kingdom and the United States, even Dubai, so there wasn't
anything seedy about going there. Besides, it was good for the Government.
You see, if takings are, say, Rs50 lakhs, then the government gets Rs20 lakhs
of it in tax. And then any of the remaining Rs30 lakhs that gets paid out in
winnings—if you win over a certain amount—are also taxed, about thirty-
five percent I think, so the government ends up with more than half of the
takings." A day at the races, as Das describes it, was a legitimate and inex-
pensive way to pass one's time: it was not about gambling or accruing debt.

"It was harder to win in Madras than in other places," he went on, "not
because there was more cheating . . . that's not the right way to put it. But
there was more fixing of races, I think, so it was harder to work out who
might win just by studying the form, you needed inside information too. But
I didn't make a loss there, I think I probably broke even on bets. No, the

problem with Madras, apart from the fixing, was that the facilities were not as good as elsewhere. The canteen food wasn't even up to much, it cost more on the gate to get in, and it would get so packed out you could hardly move. But you didn't have to go to the place itself to play. If it was, say, the Deccan Derby in Hyderabad, which takes place on October 2, or the Bangalore Kingfisher Derby, you could go to other race courses, bet, and watch the race live on television screens."

His favorite venue for the races, he told me, was the Mahalaxmi race course in what was then Bombay, a course I was familiar with as it was visible from the station where Anandapuram villagers away begging had set up camp, and where we attended two meetings in 2011. "Again, I didn't go there often, but if I was in Bombay for some other business, perhaps, I might go there. I didn't know about this kind of thing when I was living on Dadar station, but I visited, years later, with friends from that time. The travel agent friend who helped me when I was first on the station, Gopi, he took me there once, in the late 1990s it must have been I think. We went in at about 10am, bought our books to study the form, and did our calculations. It won't always work, studying the odds and the form: a good horse might come down half way around the race, and that will really change what's expected to happen. So it's a gamble, but we can manage the risks a bit. We'd study the books and then, in the last five minutes before the race starts, we'd place our bets."

Although Das had initially been reticent about talking about horse racing, now that he had started, he became increasingly more animated. "Sometimes we'd play to win, sometimes each way, and sometimes we'd play doubles, jackpots and so on—lots of types of bets! Once, I went to Bombay with Rs3,000, and I played the super jackpot on that first day: it meant I had to back a winner in all six races to win anything. So I selected my races, and put on Rs1,920, backing several horses in some of the races to make sure I got a win." My grasp of the complex mathematical calculations was lost at this point in the story, but the upshot of the bet was that Das's final horse was a mafia group owned horse named "Nothing Better," and he won, bagging Das around Rs10,000. "I bought a book for the next day, went to a lodge and booked a room for Rs400. I'd been staying with our begging people, sleeping outside—'why unnecessarily waste money on a room?' I'd thought—but now I'd got Rs10,000 in my pocket, so why not!? It's also safer, with that much money. I washed my clothes in the sink, had a good bath, and, feeling refreshed, lay down on the bed and studied the book. The next day came, and again I went and put Rs1,920 on a super jackpot bet. And I won all of them again! This time I won a net total of Rs30,000! Now, Bombay isn't a cheap place to be, and I probably spent another Rs6,000 at the race course—a few side bets I didn't win, some beers, and food. But that meant I still had Rs34,000 profit from the two days to take back home."

On that occasion, the money apparently went into paying some of his outstanding debts. "I wouldn't usually make that sort of money," he conceded, "but I had a big win one other time on the Bombay races, betting from the course in Vijayawada. Nineteen ninety-seven I think it was. I paid out Rs75,000 in taxes! I came back with a total of Rs1.13lakhs, and I had a lot of debts at that time, so I was able to repay a whole lot of them off all at once. I didn't tell people where the money had come from, and they weren't interested anyway. They just wanted it back. I showed the winning slips to my father, I think, to assure him that he didn't need to worry so much about our debts. That time they paid me by check: I'd played in Vijayawada, and because the manager there didn't have the power to sign checks for that much, he had to send a note to Hyderabad. I had to go there myself to pick up the check, and once I'd deposited it in the bank it took two months to clear, so we lost a lot of interest that could have been building up on it! But then I paid Rs55,000 to Wesley, and we spent Rs20,000 in the house—new saris, clothes, a visit to my mother's place in Madras—and paid others back as well."

It was harder to get Das to talk about losses, but there were a few: "Sometimes it's very horrible," he said. "You might put Rs10,000 on a horse and win ten times that in one race, then put all that money on another horse, a dead cert, and lose it by a hair's breadth. It's happened. I'm not saying it's happened to me, but it does happen to people all the time. The thing to do, if you've got Rs2 lakhs, is to put just ten percent of it—Rs20,000—on one side for betting with. I know people who live like that. They'll draw the Rs20,000 for the day from their accounts, and place the money on safe bets. If they make Rs6,000 profit on the first Rs10,000, then they stop. Rs6,000 is a good return for one day, no? If not, he'll play the remaining Rs10,000. If that's lost, okay, he'll stop for the day and try again tomorrow. But overall he can make a good living that way. If you're betting each way and will get something on each of the first three or four places, as long as you're playing safe bets you should win most of the time. Play like that two or three times a week and you're in a comfortable position."

Although Das presents betting on the horses as a profitable affair, the fact that he has nothing to show for his big wins—and that he already had such big debts to pay off in 1997 when, a year earlier, he had been handed the money to clear his slate—suggests to me that he preferred not to recall his losses. I can also now see why, for someone whose salary always seems too low to meet basic needs, gambling appears to be a plausible response. If you anyway cannot pay the rice bill, why not place the whole lot on a horse and hope for the best? If it loses, you still won't be able to pay the rice bill; if it wins, you can pay your dues and more besides. As your debts soar to amounts that you never have any chance of paying—even if you hand over your entire salary each month—then the impulse to take a chance becomes even greater. And when the racecourse not only offered that chance but an escape from the seemingly inescapable demands of the colony members around him, its allure becomes almost irresistible.

The stresses of the job were starting to manifest themselves elsewhere in Das's life, too. Although he had always avoided alcohol during these years working on the station, in the decade he had lived in Anandapuram he had begun to indulge in the occasional tipple. "But it never became a habit until much later on," he insists, "not until after 1997 at least. My first drink though, that must have been when I was at a meeting with Emma somewhere, in Hyderabad, I think, and we went to someone's house—they were Roman Catholics—and we were offered a drink. I'd already seen, on that training course, that respectable people sometimes took a drink, and foreigners do too, so sometimes I'd have one if I was offered. But not much."

When I was in Anandapuram in 1996, and went with Das and a couple of his colleagues to sell bags and table linen to Americans living at the hill station of Kodaikanal, I remember us having a drink. It was cold and wet in Kodai, and we were staying in damp, whitewashed rooms in a lodge fairly near the centre of town. Alcohol, as the local doctor always told me, was considered essential for warmth in cold climates, and so we shared bottles of Kingfisher beer, fortified with Indian whisky. As we had only one or two glasses in the room between four or five of us, we took it in turns to drink, downing the amber liquid as quickly as possible for maximum impact and to free up the glass for the next person. Another of Das's colleagues, Gurumurthy, once told me that "sipping drinks, as you call it, I think, is popular in your culture, I've seen it in American films. But it's not what we do here. We need to complete the drinks as soon as possible and then we go on to eat afterwards."[4] Alcohol was also prohibited in Andhra Pradesh at that time, which is why the opportunity to drink while we were in Kodai—which is in Tamil Nadu—was one to savour. Given the chance, Das took part in such rituals. His point, though, was that he didn't feel the urgent *need* for alcohol until later on.

On occasions, drink also contributed to his problems, bringing lightly shielded tensions prematurely into the open. At the end of a fundraising cycle rally from Anandapuram to Chennai that I had taken part in—organized by Gurumurthy—Das met us and the other cyclists at a lodge he had booked for us on the city's peripheries. The plan was that we should congregate there, take rest, and then cycle to the finish line, where the press would be waiting to photograph us, early the next morning. Prohibition was still in force in Andhra Pradesh, so that evening, at Gurumurthy's insistence, we took advantage of having crossed the state borders and bought bottles of whisky and brandy to share among the cycle team. We drank furtively, huddled together in our shared room, sharing the two glasses that we had found in the bathroom. The mood was a euphoric one: we had all cycled 200 miles together over several days, and the bonds between us felt strong. There were, however, clear tensions between Das, who had arrived by train to meet us, and his deputy, Gurumurthy. Emboldened by the drink, Gurumurthy apparently accosted Das as we left the lodge to go for dinner. "I work like a dog, a *dog*, for you, and what do I get for it?" he slurred scornfully. "You know that *I* should be in your job now, not you!" Das—or so he claimed when he recounted the story to me—had ignored the provocation, tutted, and stepped aside. But the venom with which he reported it the next day, and the clarity with which he still remembered it, more than a decade later, suggested that the comments had stung him deeply. Gurumurthy, of whom he was always wary, had become another adversary.

It was also through drink, though, that Das found a third escape route from the pressures of work. He had been sitting at the front of his house one day chatting to Fauzia, one of his neighbours, while his wife was inside boiling rice. Fauzia's own husband was away, as he usually was, begging in Bombay. Das got on well with women: his manner was gentle, he was friendly and he could make them laugh. He and Fauzia were laughing about something when she pointed up to a guava hanging down from a branch of the tree above her, and said, with a smile, "Das garu, you see that guava, up there in the tree, is it good? I want to taste that." She licked her lips. "At the time, I just laughed," said Das, "she was just teasing, but I knew what she meant. Then, sometime later that evening, I think there had been a fight or some tension in the house—maybe between Elizabeth Rani and Mariya, I can't remember—and troubles in the office, so I went out and bought a quarter bottle of whisky and drank it right down. I bought another one and came straight back to our street. The drink made me very bold: I knew her husband wasn't there and her daughter was out somewhere, so I just walked straight into the house and sat down on the bed. She smiled at me and said, 'Ah, so you've come to try that guava, have you?' Then I started to touch her, and we ended up having sex. That was the first time I had experience with anyone else other than Mariya in Anandapuram. But we didn't want an affair, just a taste. It only happened now and then."

There were other encounters during that period, but they were all one-off, brief affairs. Another of Das's neighbours, a leprosy-affected man called Sambaiah, had asked him to accompany him and his wife to a hospital for some leprosy-related treatment. The bridge of his nose had entirely collapsed, and he was keen to obtain a prosthetic bridge that would make him look more like he once had. "We went to the hospital," Das reported, "and we finished the initial job, of getting him admitted, in half an hour or so. Sambaiah needed to stay there until that evening, though, or maybe even the next day, and so he told me and his wife that we'd may as well travel back to the Colony. But as we left the hospital, Estheramma, his wife, said to me, 'I'm not feeling well now, let's take some rest here first and then go.' And so we went to a lodge nearby, got a room, and she wanted to take sleep. And I said, 'Look, I am a man, how can we be here together in the same room alone and rest on the bed?' But I was away from the colony, so I felt free, and I knew that I was cured of leprosy and couldn't do any harm to anyone, that I could enjoy sex and all. So I finally agreed to her suggestion that we shared a room, and we had a meal there and a bath, and then we had sex. After that we left there at 7 o'clock, and I brought her home. But again, this wasn't a proper affair: she was younger than her husband and had lots of other contacts. I think he used to be rough with her, especially because he knew what she was like, but now he leaves it and doesn't bother."

There were other encounters, too, details of which trickled out slowly over the course of our interviews. No sooner had he assured me that there were no further affairs to report than he would be reminded of another. But there were, to my certain knowledge, at least three more sexual liaisons in the village, all of them one-off events. In every case he described, Das was presented as a passive recipient of the women's advances: they were portrayed as pulling him into their houses, pinning him against the wall, and then hoisting up their saris and petticoats. "What can I do? I'm a man," he said, shrugging his shoulders.

All these incidents, he recalled, happened sometime after my own departure from the village in September 1996. Until then, despite being pessimistic that anything could ever really be changed in how people in the village thought and behaved, he appeared to have things, at least in the workplace, more or less under control. The difficulties were mounting, however. While I was in the colony, for example, Das was forced to take the decision to close the synthetic diamond-cutting unit that had, until then, employed around twelve people. Although closure of the unit did not quite cause the uproar we feared it might, it was unsettling for people, particularly as money in other projects was also scarce, and there had been no proper review of staff wages and salaries for a long time. In the past, there had always been something new going on. There was the massive house building scheme in the late 1980s, followed by the construction of a new school and clinic, a large work unit that had housed the office, the weaving and sewing areas, the gem cutting room and the plastics welding unit, and then, in 1994, the building of a new, stand-alone office, complete with meeting rooms. As long as things were happening, not only was the hope of more and better paid jobs kept alive, but the large amounts of income coming in for capital building projects also helped to bridge gaps in other areas of expenditure. With Emma gone and building complete, there was a danger that things were looking as though they were stagnating.

NOTES

1. See, for discussion of the approaches taken by NGOs, Katy Gardner and David Lewis, *Anthropology, Development and the Post-modern Challenge* (London: Pluto Press, 1996); and Johan Pottier, ed., *Practising Development: Social Science Perspectives* (London: Routledge, 1993).

2. In thinking through this particular dispute, which I analyze in more detail elsewhere (Staples, *Peculiar People*), I drew inspiration from Jonathan Spencer, *A Sinhala Village in a Time of Trouble: Politics and Change in Rural Sri Lanka* (New Delhi: Oxford University Press, 2000).

3. For a more detailed discussion of this relationship see James Staples, "Becoming a man: personhood and masculinity in a south Indian leprosy colony," *Contributions to Indian Sociology* 39, 2 (2005): 279–305.

4. See also Alter, *Knowing Dildas*, 55. He notes, of local Himalyan liquor, that "It is not in the least like a cocktail. You drink it down as fast as possible, a tumbler full at a time, and then relish the effect."

Chapter Eight

The Fall . . .

From the outside looking in, things were going reasonably well in the year after Das had taken over in Anandapuram. As if to celebrate the colony's resilience in the face of change, the end of 1996 was marked, thanks to a last minute donation, with a communal meal, served on narrow Krishna-blue tables, under brightly patterned canopies to protect diners from the late winter sun. Despite fears that donations would dry up without a foreigner to account for them the other programs were all still running, too. There were orders coming in for the weaving unit; the coconut, sappota and cashew nut trees nurtured by those on the custodial care scheme were at last bearing fruit; and, after years of waiting, government recognition of the colony's elementary school finally appeared to be in the offing. Early in 1997, the community also won a bid, which Das and I had drawn up via email, for funding to extend the weaving unit and to create at least ten new jobs. Rereading newsletters produced by Anandapuram's UK charity for that period, the mood in Anandapuram seemed decidedly upbeat.

That was what such newsletters were for: to reassure supporters that it was business as usual, and that the more they gave, the more could be achieved. But from Das's perspective it was in 1997 that things seriously started to become unravelled. The signs were there from the start. On January 1, only a few hours after the debris of the celebratory meal had been cleared away, the Elders marked the occasion by showing a video of a play previously recorded by members of the community. They had hired a large television set and a video cassette player for precisely that purpose, and it had been set up outside the community hall. A public film showing, or even a live performance from a travelling theatre company, was not uncommon in the village, particularly at festival times when everyone had returned from begging trips. Unlike many of the Elders' decisions, this one did not appear particularly controversial. However, in this case a young man called Nathaniel, the healthy son of leprosy-affected parents, performed the lead role in the play.

I had known Nathaniel from previous trips to the village: after training as a fitter, he had worked in the synthetic gem-cutting unit that Das had closed, and, young and newly-wed, could often be found in the early evenings hanging out with his peers, playing badminton or carrom board, or taking snacks in the teashops. Compared to many of his wiry contemporaries he was well-built; one of the shiniest examples of the nutritional success of a long running school meals program in the village. It was because he seemed so fit and healthy that his death, just a few months earlier, had been such a shock to everyone concerned, myself included. According to a letter Das wrote to me at the time, Nathaniel had visited the office to apply for a loan to start up his own business. When he fell ill a couple of days later, the local doctor referred him to hospital to be treated for what appeared to be a minor kidney infection. He died on the cycle rickshaw on the way to the hospital.

The play was produced shortly before Nathaniel died, and until now had not been publicly screened. Nathaniel's widow, seeing her late husband projected on the screen without prior warning, was upset. No-one had asked her or her family whether they minded the video being played. She pushed to the front of the crowd and yelled at Gopalkrishnan, then President of the Elders. "Who are you to show my husband without any permission? Without even a word to us?" She was angry, and her voice was raised. Consumption of alcohol was common among the men at festival times, and Gopalkrishnan, who in any case liked to drink, had been downing arrack since the feast, and was staggering perilously across the stage. Waving his arms toward her dismissively, he told her that she should go away, leave the audience to watch the video and enjoy the celebration in peace. Who was she to tell them what they could and could not show?

It was the provocation that the widow's brother, Daniel, had been waiting for. Daniel was one of the young men who had previously lost his job for his role in setting up the Youth Welfare Society and campaigning for the Telugu Desam Party, and although he had been reinstated there remained considerable tension between him and the Elders. His victory had left the Elders bitter and Daniel emboldened. He joined his sister at the front in calling for the film to be switched off and, in the ensuing argument about whether or not the film would be played, he was reported to have pushed Gopalkrishnan to the ground and, to the greater consternation of those who had gathered to watch, had knocked over the large television set that had been hired for the occasion.

Das had not been present at the showing that evening. Whenever the office was closed he took the opportunity to slip away, to Tradefair in Chennai where he still felt respected, to the races or to watch a film in peace. On this occasion, he said he had spent the evening at the cinema in Vijayawada, two hours away on an express train. Nevertheless, it did not take long for him to find out what had happened: both the President and Secretary of the Elders turned up at his house early next morning, and were there waiting on the bed outside when he emerged, in vest and lunghi, from the inside room. "They said that Daniel had tried to beat them, and that this was against all the colony rules and regulations," Das recalled. "He had beaten an office bearer, they told me, so we needed to remove him from his job. I told them to calm down, and that they'd need to come to the office to talk about it properly."

They gave Das time to wash at the water pump in front of his house, dress and drink the tea his wife had been preparing when they called, and then he went to the office to meet the full Elders' committee. He could sense the anger that was building up. "I said to them, 'Look, it didn't happen here in the workplace, so we need to be careful. Yes, Daniel's a troublemaker, we know that, but because of that we also need to do things properly.' I recommended that we should first give him a warning letter, and then suspend him from his job while we look into what happened. Only if we do that, and follow the proper procedures, should we dismiss him. After what happened the time before, I told them we had to stop and think before throwing people out of their jobs."

The Elders, and particularly the President, whose status had been threatened by such a public act against him, were in no mood for following bureaucratic processes. "They were very angry," Das remembered, "and so were lots of the older villagers who had been there and seen what happened. Forty or fifty people came to the office with them, lots of them leprosy patients who are usually away begging but were back for the new year festival, and they were demanding that Daniel should be removed from his post immediately. So I sent him a note, telling him to come and explain himself, and to tell him he was suspended while we looked into his case. It was enough to give me some time and to stop the people pressing me for action."

Daniel refused to take the letter, however, and neither did he come to the office to explain what had happened. "A week later, The Elders and others came back to office again, and said, 'okay, he hasn't responded, he's had a chance, now you need to remove him.' And I warned them then that maybe this would make problems. Office staff, people like Gurumurthy, the social worker, were all there, but they never said anything to support me! Nobody wanted to stand up to the Elders in front of them. Anyway, the Secretary was very bold. He said he didn't care if Daniel took them to court: 'We'll just collect Rs100 or whatever we need from each house and pay the costs with that,' he said, and I could tell they weren't interested in the consequences. So what could I do? The pressure was coming from them, I had no support, so finally I signed a letter telling Daniel that he had been dismissed and had it sent to him."

Although the full consequences of dismissing Daniel did not start to become apparent for another year or so, in the short term it helped to fuel what until then had only been vague plans among the workforce to set up a trade union. Like the Youth Welfare Society before it—now moribund, but still lurking in the background, biding its time—the union was a response by under-represented groups within the village to their feeling that their concerns were being ignored. The office management, as the union's founder members expressed it, had little capacity to resist the excesses of the Elders, and Daniel's case made this plain. The workers—tailors, weavers, gardeners and clinic ward boys among them—were already becoming restless. Daniel's dismissal just spurred them on. A review of their salary scales had been due when Emma left in 1995, but they were still waiting for the Management Committee to discuss the issue and make a decision two years on.

"These white people had come here with their pious ways," one of the founder members of the union told me some years later, "and then they abandoned us to a bunch of thieves. What do you do in that situation?" The "thieves" to whom he referred included the Elders, or at least some of them, and the office staff. "When the office staff went out on business they took big advances to cover their expenses," one of the tailors, another founder of the union, once complained to me, "but they never paid their balances back straight away. Then they'd go on another trip, take another advance, and the same thing would happen. Some of them owed a fortune to the office. But if we took any advances on our salaries, the cashier would deduct the full amount when we got paid. It was unfair. We kept sending notes to the management committee, asking them to look at how much money office staff owed, but nothing seemed to be changing." They had a point: all senior staff, Das especially, owed the office substantial sums of money.

When complaints about salaries or other matters came from individuals, wearing though this was, Das could usually fob them off. But now they had come together as a trade union, affiliated to the All India Trade Union Congress (AITUC), they were much more powerful: another interest group to balance against the demands of the Elders, the management committee, Gurumurthy, and the people he worked with in the office on a day-to-day basis. He probably knew, for example, that he should be stricter at getting colleagues to settle their accounts, but it was only by turning a blind eye that his own failures to return advances were not made even more public than they already were. "Anyway, I wasn't stealing anything," he told me, defensively. "It was all there in the accounts books; you could see how much everyone owed. I wasn't deceiving any one. But if I didn't have the money to pay back, what could I do? I knew I'd have to wait until later."

Das's attempts to find money to pay off various moneylenders were becoming increasingly desperate. As it emerged a couple of years later when I was in the village doing fieldwork, at one point he had asked his friend Venkata Reddy to cash one of his chit funds and lend him Rs10,000 to keep his creditors at bay. Venkata Reddy obliged, but when he urgently needed the money himself—to cover the medical expenses of one of his nephews—Das borrowed the money from the office, signing it out as an advance to Venkata Reddy. It was because neither he nor Venkata Reddy were entitled to such advances that details of the transaction eventually came out—first through village gossip, later at management committee meetings.

As things got harder to juggle in the work place, Das found little comfort at home. "Mariya, she doesn't know anything, so how could I talk to her about my problems?" he said bitterly when I asked why he didn't discuss what was going on with her. Perhaps, I had suggested, she could have been a sounding board, someone who, whether she understood or not, could at least be trusted not to gossip about what he told her. "You knew, did you, that Mariya also had a drinking habit?" he interrupted me, his thoughts now directed firmly towards the domestic sphere. I had not known for sure, although I had heard the rumors. According to Das, it started to become a problem when they had moved out of his father's house into their own. "She'd originally got the habit from her mother, though: she would have given her *kallu* [palm toddy] to drink as a child—it was common in those days, in villages. But after we moved into our own place, sometimes I would bring home alcohol for me to drink to forget my problems: a bottle of beer, sometimes, or more often a quarter bottle of brandy or whisky. I might drink one at the shop and bring another back with me, to help me to sleep later on. After a while, sometimes it would just disappear! Someone might call me outside to talk about a work problem, so I'd leave it there on a shelf inside, and when I returned to the house a bit later the bottle would be gone. At first I thought she was hiding them to stop me drinking. Sometimes she'd say that the bottle had fallen over and smashed. But I realized later she had been drinking it herself! And it got to the point where if there was no drink in the evening she wouldn't eat. We'd have fights over it. She'd demand that I go and buy some. She'd weep. So I'd have to go out on my bicycle and buy it for her."

Life in the village was difficult for Mariya too. Although moving into their own house meant she no longer had to suffer Elizabeth Rani's insults at close quarters, it also meant she spent much more of her time alone with their young son, particularly as her husband's departures to Vijayawada or Chennai were becoming more frequent. Their house, barely furnished and seldom with more provisions than were required to meet immediate needs, was not much of a haven for her either, particularly at the low points when they had failed to pay the electricity bill and there was no light or fan or when, during the monsoon, water dripped down into one corner of the main room. They did have a second-hand television (one of eighty or so in the village at the time) bought with a loan, but little else: a couple of wonky string beds, a decrepit kerosene stove rather than the gas rings others were now investing in, and a few metal trunk boxes for their clothes and cooking pots. The fact that Das, the highest paid officer in the colony, also had one of the scruffiest houses was something that others commented on often: "Where do you think his money goes?" Gurumurthy once asked me, casually but mischievously, watching me from the corner of his eye to see how I might respond. "Some of us wonder if he's building another house somewhere or if he has another family."

I do not know whether Mariya entertained such thoughts: she probably had more prosaic concerns. Other wives might have taken solace in the company of the other women in the street, in their lovers or in the church, but none of these options seemed to appeal much to Mariya. She had always been shy and insecure and, according to Das, was consequently quick to take offence at comments from the women who lived close by. "Sometimes," Das said, "I'd come back to the house and find that she and another woman in the street were arguing, and I'd say to Mariya, 'Be quiet, go in the house or I'll beat you!' Not that I did beat her, but I wanted her to stop. I can say that to her, as my wife, but I can't say it to the other woman. That's up to her husband. But she'll say, 'Oh, why you supporting her, not me?' and get even more upset. We'd quite often have that kind of fight."

Under such circumstances, perhaps it was not surprising that Mariya also used liquor to take the edge off her sorrows, while Das took the same route to postponing his own. "There was no other solution for me at that time," he said. "I had family pressures on one side, all these other problems on the other. Other people in my place would definitely have committed suicide or gone mad. In the daytime, when I came home from the office, I'd take my mind off everything by playing with Joshua and the other children in the street, or when I woke up in the middle of the night I'd switch on the television and try to distract my mind. It wasn't easy."

Another reason for Mariya's drinking escalating at around the time it did might have been because it was also sometime in 1997 that Das's most significant love affair, with a women called Padma, began. "It wasn't like with the others," Das said. "When I went into Fauzia's house and had sex with her it was like in the old days in Bombay when I visited Grant Road. It was just for relief, for fun. But with Padma it was different. There was a real affection between us, and she wanted us to be together, like a real family."

It all began one evening when he was coming back from one of his escapist trips to Vijayawada. "I think I'd been to see a film or something, I can't really remember," he told me, "and, as usual, I'd got up on a berth and slept for a while. I woke up when we were about an hour away from our stop, and I saw her sitting there on the seat below. There was a seat free next to her, and she patted it for me to sit down next to her." Although Das did not know Padma particularly well at the time, he knew who she was. Her husband worked as a peon and cleaner in the office. She was closer in age to Das than his wife; plump and outgoing; and unlike most women in the village she was overtly Hindu. "Lots of people are on the inside," she once confided in me, "but I'm the only one bold enough to say so openly!" A large poster of Lord Venkateswara—an incarnation of Vishnu—was pasted above her front door, and a laminated photograph of the orange clad, afro-haired guru Satya Sai Babu was perched prominently on the top of her television set.

"I sat there next to her," Das went on with his story, "and gradually we began to talk, just in a general way. She told me that her husband's relatives lived in Vijayawada, and that she had been to visit them. Soon, she dozed off to sleep herself and, in her sleep, her arm moved across and she touched me on the knee. Then suddenly she woke up, looked shocked that she had her hand on me, and quickly moved it away. 'Is she pretending or is it real?' I thought to myself, but I didn't say anything. I wasn't sure. Then she said, 'Oh Das, I am so very fed up with my life! I get no satisfaction from my husband. He is always titillating me, coming in to the bathroom and watching me take my clothes off to bathe, but then he leaves without touching me. I want to be a proper wife!'"

"But because she can't—because her husband can't, I don't think, actually have sex with her—she says that she wants to have a friendship with another man. I am a Brahmin man, and she is also some kind of Brahmin I think; she's from Orissa. Maybe she also thinks that I am a senior person, I have a good job in the colony, and that she doesn't want to have a relationship with someone of lower status. So I shrug—what can I do?—and I say, 'okay, I will meet you in the next week.'"

"When the time came she was very bold. I had forgotten about that day until you asked me, but I was about to go to the bazaar, to get some shopping I think, and she called me over and said, 'I am going to Vijayawada now, you need to come.' As straightforwardly as that! So I said back, 'Okay, I will come with you,' like that. And off we went to Vijayawada. She was supposed to be going to her husband's relatives' place, but she had said to them that she needed to go to this and that temple first and that she would come later. And, you know, not a single paise did I spend, that's the truth of it. She had some money with her, so we went to a hotel, and we booked a room. She wanted us to be a high-up officer and his wife, to live that kind of life. She dressed beautifully like some kind of merchant caste lady, and she wanted me also to be like a big man, like a gentleman. Later on, she'd ask me to wear good clothes and other things. But that time, we went to the room, we had sex together, and then we went to a meals hotel, where we ordered some middle class type dishes, not the kind of meals we'd usually have. We had chapattis, vegetable curries, naan bread, that kind of thing: the sort of food you get served in a three-star hotel. And then she said, 'okay, let's go to the cinema,' and so we did, and she was very happy. She looked at me and said: 'Oh, don't leave me or I will die!' Then we stayed together in the hotel that night. When we woke up, she went to her relatives, and I took the train back to Anandapuram, and I went to work."

For Padma, the affair allowed her to live out a fantasy; to be someone other than a leprosy patient in a leprosy colony, cooking and cleaning for a husband who was not sexually interested in her. It gave her an excuse to dress in her finest saris, to sample the luxuries of middle class life. For Das, it offered moments of respite from the problems at work and at home that otherwise threatened to suffocate him. Away from all of that, lying next to Padma in their hotel room in Vijayawada, he could finally sleep at night. In his house in the colony he slept only fitfully, worries about his growing debts and other pressures awakening him at regular intervals throughout the night.

Das was not sure when Mariya became aware of his affair with Padma. She never confronted him directly but, later on, if he had to go away over night, sometimes she would make comments along the lines of: "So, is *she* there already, waiting for you?" Even at the start, though, she was irked by his regular and prolonged departures: Das was seldom at home at weekends and often organized his work trips to allow for an overnight stay away, giving her ample opportunity to drink alone. If he was not in Vijayawada with Padma he would often spend weekends in Chennai, sleeping on Trade-fair's floor and using brief business meetings as an excuse for staying away from Friday until Monday.

All things considered, it was remarkable that, unbeknownst to her until later, Mariya fell pregnant with her second child in early 1998. "She never had much interest in sex," Das said, adding, with a bashful chuckle: "If I told her I'd give her something she wanted—a new sari, perhaps—then she might concede, but it would only be once in every two or three months, and some-times there might be a gap of six months even."

Mariya stopped drinking altogether, either just before or soon after she became pregnant. "She was sick," Das recalled, "she'd been drinking one night and she complained that the room was going round and round, and that some devils had possessed her. I took her to the doctor, he said that she was very anemic, that her nerves were also bad, and that if she continued to drink alcohol she would die. She was terrified by that remark. She completely stopped from that moment. Now she doesn't even like the smell."

As their second child began to grow in Mariya's tiny belly, the problems Das had predicted when the Elders demanded Daniel's dismissal started to take shape. Bolstered by the support of the union, Daniel again engaged a lawyer and took the organization and Das, whose name was on the letter from the courts, to civil court for unfair dismissal. Das also blamed Daniel for encouraging the union to pursue a case for higher wages under minimum wage legislation, which also went through the courts. "The costs were just too high to pay what the law demanded," Das told me, complaining that most businesses anyway ignored the law, paying off the labor officer if he showed up unexpectedly. "We already had to pay for their health care in the clinic, to fund the school, meals for the elderly. Each family was given its own house. They got all these benefits, so we couldn't afford to pay higher salaries."

And there began what Das described as seven years of bad times; bad times which even the birth of his second child—a daughter, named Kaveri after his own sister—on September 26, 1998 could not mitigate. Indeed, in his telling of the story, Kaveri's arrival becomes conflated with all the other things that were going wrong, sometimes even cited as the cause of them. "Of course, I love my daughter," Das said hurriedly, "but it wasn't the same as when Joshua was born. At that time I was still popular in the village, and there was lots of love and affection for our family from our neighbours. Mariya was feeling elated because she had son, and my father got better when everyone had thought he was going to die. So we felt Joshua had brought us good luck."

"But after Kaveri was born, everything went wrong: money problems, the office, everything. Now, I don't really believe in palmists and astrologers and those kinds of things. But sometimes, things can bring us luck or bad luck, I think. I am not even *fully* believing in that, but if there are connections, there are connections. And I felt that Kaveri's birth brought us bad luck." Prone to ailments, from stomach upsets to high fevers, he also saw her as an additional drain on the family's scarce resources. At around the same time, his own mother, living alone now with her increasingly frail cousin, Parvathi, had a fall at her home in Chennai, and he was worried about what might become of her if she outlived Parvathi. Mariya's mother, too, had been sick and needed treatment, and she expected assistance: "They saw me as a big man compared to their own sons," Das said of his in-laws, "and so this was another burden. How could we turn away her own mother? Mariya wouldn't have let me."

As a consequence of all this, Kaveri's arrival was not greeted with quite the air of celebration that Joshua's had been. He had written to tell me of his son's birth straight away, but although we were conversing regularly by email at the time of his daughter's delivery, he never mentioned it until I arrived in India a year later and he told me about her amid a list of catastrophes that had befallen the family. His excuse for not mentioning her earlier was that fending off the court cases had become a full-time occupation. In fairness, his letters were also in his capacity as administrator of the colony's programs, to me as the secretary of a UK charity that raised funds for Anandapuram, so the focus was rightly on business affairs. But it did suggest that his daughter's arrival was not seen as an unadulterated source of joy.

The next year or so, in Das's account, is something of a blur: regular trips to the courts with the Elders (who demanded dinner and alcohol enroute), punctuated with weekends in Chennai or Vijayawada, to bet on the horses or to spend a night away with Padma. In Chennai, Tradefair, through which Anandapuram exported its products, continued to offer a welcome relief— not just because it took him back to Tamil Nadu, but also because there he was respected without having burdens placed upon him. Tradefair, as Das saw it, recognized his qualities and Vibulananthan, its idiosyncratic chief, had an uncharacteristic soft spot for Das. Perhaps it was because he also faced pressures from member organizations and his own board of trustees, and he recognized Das as the loyal ally that he was.

The management committee back in Anandapuram heard all the rumors: that Das was gallivanting around the country with the Elders in the Colony's jeep, spending all the money that could be spent on increasing salaries on drink and other pleasures. They had, on several occasions, passed resolutions to sell the jeep altogether, in the hope that visits to the court house on the bus or train would be less appealing. "They told me I shouldn't go, that I should just send our lawyer," Das told me, "but it was my name on all the papers, so I had to be there, no? I had to hear what case was being made against me."

He also, he claimed, told the committee that he needed someone else to work alongside him, to manage all the correspondence and the day-to-day activities of the staff. He could continue, he said, to do the work he had done previously: to keep and manage the accounts, and to ensure the statutory paperwork was all kept up to date but he could not do all those things *and* manage the Elders and the staff. The committee, already concerned that all was not well, agreed that something had to be done. A local doctor on the committee, long since associated with the nearby mission hospital, suggested that his own brother, Raj Kumar, who had recently returned to the area from missionary work with tribal people in Nagaland, might be well-suited for the job. Raj Kumar was available, lived close by, and had no fear of people affected by leprosy. A few doubts were expressed by other committee members, some of whom would have preferred advertising the post, but they were also aware that things could not stay as they were: Das looked set to have a nervous breakdown and they decided that appointing Raj Kumar was better than the alternative.

The next time I saw Das was in late 1999. I had travelled by train from Delhi to Vijayawada, and he came to meet me there to accompany me on the last leg of the journey to Anandapuram: a couple of hours by car. The jeep had still not been sold, but had broken down and was gathering dust in its shed alongside the colony's kitchen. Das had hired a local driver with an Ambassador car for the journey, and we bumped along in the back as it ploughed through the potholes. I was pleased to see him: it had been three years since my last visit and I was excited at the prospect of a whole year in the village to carry out fieldwork for my PhD project. Das was also keen to brief me on relations with the new project co-ordinator, which, it soon became apparent, were not good. "I thought I couldn't cope with the work because I wasn't good enough or well-educated," he told me, "but this man is much worse. All he wants to do is to sit behind a big desk."

Das's other major complaint was that Raj Kumar had "caste feeling."

I was surprised. "But he's from a very low caste, isn't he? Madiga or Mala? How could he have caste feeling?"

"I mean he's only interested in talking to those from his own group, and he favors them rather than treating us all equally," Das replied. "He tells the office staff nothing—we never know where he is, what he's doing, nothing! But then he stands outside the office in the street chatting freely to the gardeners, who also happen to be Madigas. They address him using the familiar form of 'you,' not in the polite terms they should use for speaking to their boss. We all notice it."

Invoking 'caste feeling'—especially in this inverted form—struck me, a fledgling anthropologist, as particularly interesting. When I heard it used by others it was usually by members of lower castes to discredit those who considered themselves superior; here, it was being used conversely by a Brahmin to complain—without incurring blame on himself—about his scheduled caste boss. "But aren't there others in the office from his caste background?" I said, knowing that at least one of those Raj Kumar was accused of ignoring was also a Madiga. Das shrugged off my question: "Yes, yes, maybe, but mainly he only talks to his own people. And he's also supportive of those trade union fellows, the main troublemakers. He goes and talks to them too, away from the office, on the empty space behind the clinic. And he insists on doing *all* the purchasing himself: even if we need a pencil he goes to the bazaar *himself* to buy it! What sort of project co-ordinator is this!?"

At the time, I put Das's complaints down to the difficulty of adjusting to being not in charge any longer and having to work with a new boss; that, and a need to get his defence in ahead of any accusations that Raj Kumar or others might make about him when we reached Anandapuram. Certainly, this was part of it. But over the next few weeks, despite going to great pains to avoid becoming embroiled in office politics in a way that would compromise my fieldwork, it became clear that since his appointment Raj Kumar had done little to resolve the problems he inherited. Out of his depth, and unsupported by a mostly hostile staff, he barricaded himself in the inner office when he was in the colony, and, as Das had said, seldom returned from lunch in the afternoons. Whereas Das used whisky, Padma or trips "out of station" as his retreats, Raj Kumar had his own house beyond the perimeters of the colony to withdraw to.

Despite his apparently good intentions, it became evident how far removed Raj Kumar was from the running of the organization when, in mid-November, Anandapuram's management was summoned for its annual meeting with a major European donor in the offices of a local evangelical NGO, Spreading the Word of Christ (SWC). Mr Klausman, the octogenarian bene- factor and millionaire businessman, came to India once a year, sanctioning funds to be channelled through SWC, which he funded and worked with closely. SWC, Das told me, had built an air-conditioned guesthouse specifi- cally to accommodate Mr Klausman and his wife on their visits. Anandapu- ram relied heavily on Klausman's support: his charity funded the meals program for the elderly and a welfare program for those who no longer wanted to go begging but who were not fit for full-time work, so their annual pitch to him was an important one. Klausman had only visited the colony once or twice, but he had been very taken by it and wanted to help. The colony's relationship with SWC, on the other hand, was more fraught: the NGO ran its own leprosy colonies, within which residents were more tightly controlled, and its director, John Paul, did not approve of the hands-off, and overly secular way in which Anandapuram's programs were run.

Previously, Das had attended the meetings with a couple of office staff and the main office bearers of the Elders' committee. This year, Raj Kumar and I joined them. A group of us, plus the driver, set off in a hired car, meeting up with Das and one of the office clerks, who had travelled there ahead of us by train—outside the guesthouse. Although it was in a dusty side street, behind a nondescript doorway hidden amid a row of tyre shops, the inside of the building was relatively sumptuous: air-conditioned with wood panelled walls; the scent of sandalwood incense blocking out the smells of the street; and a glass fronted fridge in the main meeting room, well-stocked with glass bottles of soft drinks and mineral water. SWC guards prevented us from entering the building, initially, but once Klausman's assistant Hans arrived, he recognized Das and called for us to come in. We were left waiting for a while in an ante-chamber, and were eventually ushered into the main meeting room, where we were offered soft drinks. A china plate of Marie biscuits was placed on the teapoy in front of us, and the Elders began eating. Raj Kumar had slipped away somewhere before this point—"to speak to his SWC friends outside," Das speculated—but Das anyway seemed happy to lead discussions about the budget. Klausman knew him well from previous meetings, and appeared pleased to see him: smiling, shaking his hand, clutch- ing on to Das's leg as he spoke. Despite his benign, rather doddery air, Klausman was aware of the tensions between Anandapuram and SWC.

"Tell me, how is Anandapuram's relationship these days with SWC?" he asked.

"What can I say? How can I possibly comment?" said Das with a shrug and a polite laugh. "Only you will know what John Paul might be saying about us!"

"He tells me that Anandapuram people are still going begging."

"*Very* few these days sir, very few. When we started, maybe there were one thousand people going begging. We've cut that by 90 percent. Only one hundred or so people go out begging these days. But how can we stop them completely? They have debts and other things to pay and their incomes are not high. But ninety percent down—we are making progress!"

"But begging's not good, no? Begging is not a good way for any human being to make a living. What dignity can any man have from begging?"

As they spoke—Das carefully responding to each of Klausman's questions and comments, politely but warmly—Klausman peered through his spectacles at the budget proposal he had been presented with. "Hmmm, you know your figures, don't you my friend?" he said to Das finally, turning to me and adding: "This man, he's very good, knows his stuff!" He looked around for Hans and signalled for him to pass a pen, which he used to write "sanctioned" across the page and sign it. He passed it back to Hans. "Thank you sir!" Das beamed, satisfied at a job well done. I was seeing him at his best.

At that moment, as if to highlight the contrast between the two men, Raj Kumar burst in, apologizing for his lateness. I had forgotten, until then, that he was even with us, and was suddenly struck by the extent he had been excluded—or had excluded himself—from the whole transaction. "Who is this?" asked Klausman, peering above his spectacles, brow furrowed. With a flicker of satisfaction passing across his face, Das replied: "Oh, this is Raj Kumar. He does some of the correspondence for us and a few other things." Raj Kumar stretched forward and put out his hand to Klausman, trying at the same time to scowl discreetly at Das. "Actually, the project chief," he said quietly, but his voice was drowned out by one of the Elders who, having downed his *Thums Up!* cola too quickly, let out a very loud burp at precisely that moment. It was the only thing the Elders contributed to the whole meeting.

The encounter successfully over and an invitation extended to us to attend SWC's church service followed by lunch, we emerged back in to the sticky midday warmth of the street. "Did you notice how Klausman had no interest in him at all?" Das asked me casually, but with barely disguised pleasure. "He's an outsider, that's why."

When we met SWC's director John Paul in the church, however, it was clear that he had a rather less rosy impression of Das than Klausman did. "Good man!" he boomed, stepping across to pat Das heartily on the back. Clad in a spotless, silky white shirt, fingers replete with bejewelled rings, he cut a smooth figure next to a rather down at heel looking Das, despite the fact that he was nearly as old as Klausman. His combed over hair was dyed jet black, and he smelt strongly of coconut oil and lavender talcum powder. An evangelical Christian from a scheduled caste, prone to shouting "Hallelujah!" at the slightest provocation, he and Das had little, beyond Klausman, in common. "Your man, I hear," he said, turning toward me and pointing towards Das. "I *also* hear that for every fifty days he spends in Anandapuram, he spends fifty days in Chennai," and, turning back to Das with a smile that revealed a perfect set of white teeth, "that's right, isn't it? What he does there I don't know!" Visibly uncomfortable, Das muttered that it was not the case. "We do a lot of exporting of our woven goods from Chennai," he said, addressing his comments to Klausman, who stood alongside John Paul. "So yes, I make a trip there now and again. But not so often. People will gossip, of course, but you mustn't believe everything you hear!"

The suggestion that Das was spending a lot of time away from Anandapuram came as no surprise to me: the village, as ever, was full of rumors about it, and, although it had not yet become openly commented upon, someone had already told me about his relationship with Padma. I also knew from experience that he was often not around if I called to see him at his house in the evenings or at the weekends. What was interesting was that, somehow, despite mounting debts to the office, court cases on all sides and his apparent inability to keep either the Elders or the staff under control, he was still able to command respect—and consequently funds for Anandapuram—from overseas donors. Maybe, having worked so closely with Emma for ten years he had learned to present himself in a way that appealed to them: unlike others I met in similar posts in NGOs, he was charming but never obsequious, and he had a dry, self-deprecating sense of humour that European visitors seemed to warm to. It was perhaps in recognition of his ability with donors that, despite gossip about his outstanding advances from the office, no one in the colony seemed to be calling for his resignation.

The same could not be said for Raj Kumar. Things came to a head when the Management Committee met in March 2000, by which time the Elders were openly calling for his dismissal. They said that he rarely came to work and, when he did, that he did not do anything useful. They were also angry with him, although they did not say so, because he refused to sanction all the expenditure they demanded, and in doing all the purchasing himself, deprived them of the paybacks from suppliers that they, and various staff members, had become accustomed to. After several hours of discussion, the committee decided that Raj Kumar would have to go.

Das, I had envisaged, would be thrilled at Raj Kumar's demise, but when he was called to the meeting later that day to be informed that a new project co-ordinator was to be appointed, and that his own job title would revert to Accounts Officer—a role he had intimated he wanted to go back to—he displayed little emotion. He seemed exhausted and past caring. I attributed his state in part to the recent death of his mother's cousin Parvathi, who his mother had lived with now for nearly thirty-five years, first in Mumbai and later in Chennai. Parvathi's sons and daughters had all left home now—all but one of them were living overseas—and her husband, the tax inspector

Subrahmanyam, had died soon after they finished building their own house in Chennai, ten years before. Since then it had been just the two women. I had visited them with Das only a couple of weeks earlier, and Parvathi, as she had been the previous time I saw her, was rocking gently to and fro on the wooden swing suspended from the ceiling in the middle of the central reception room. She was paler than the last time, but still talkative. She showed us video-tapes of one of her son's weddings and of another son's rented apartment in the Middle East, where he was working. "It's like a five star hotel!" said Das, as the camera panned over the kettle and the microwave oven in the kitchen, showing off the facilities. Parvathi's offspring had done well. Das's mother, who had doubtlessly seen the films before sat on the floor at the other end of the room, now recovered from her earlier fall, getting up whenever the older woman needed anything or, at one point, to bring us tea and snacks. "SMT we call it," Das had said, alluding again to Brahmin ways of doing things. "Sweet, *Manta* [savoury], Tea! You need to eat something sweet—like the *jalabi*, then something hot, like this salt biscuit, then we need to drink sweet tea. Everything is properly balanced then for our bodies."

We were, apparently, the last people other than Das's mother to see Parvathi alive. One of her sons, an accountant now living in the UK, had telephoned Das on his arrival back in India to tell him that Parvathi had died, peacefully. He said that the funeral rites had already been completed, and that he should not worry about his own mother. Although they would probably sell the big house his father had built, they would always take care of her. Das did not say very much about it at the time, other than to express relief that his mother would be looked after. But he stayed in Anandapuram that weekend, taking to his bed with what he claimed was "typhoid" (an upset stomach) and "malaria" (a high temperature).

With Raj Kumar gone, the project co-ordinator's post was eventually filled, in May 2000, by Dr. Johan—a Christian doctor from the local town. Dr. Johan, more commanding than his predecessor, was well received by the community. He was elderly—available to take the post because he had just retired from a more lucrative position—but unafraid of the Elders or other authority, and better able to deal with the staff than Raj Kumar had been. His style, to me, seemed overly paternalistic, and I felt uncomfortable about his public prayers to mark every eventuality. But his approach fitted a locally familiar model of management, and he seemed to have no problem in getting things done. Muttered complaints by the Secretary of the Elders that he did not listen enough to their demands seemed to me a sign that he was doing well.

In the time between Dr. Johan's appointment and his arrival in the office to take up the post, however, there had been a development in respect of the trade union's court case. The morning after Dr. Johan's interview, a payment order, demanding compensation of Rs300,000 to be paid to forty-one staff who had been underpaid according to the minimum wage legislation, arrived by courier. The court had found against the colony, according to the letter that Das read out to me and the Elders, who had been called to the office, because its representative—then Raj Kumar—had failed to appear in court when summonsed. It was at moments like this that Das seemed genuinely energized by the work; all the more so on this occasion because it allowed him to show how much more effective he was than Raj Kumar. By the time he briefed me and the Elders about what was going on he had already rung and taken advice from Cedric, their legal brief, and was gearing up to leave for the high court in Hyderabad to appeal against the finding, apparently the only action now available to them. The Elders nodded in unison: if necessary, they said, they could call people back from begging in Mumbai and stage a protest of physically disabled leprosy patients outside the court house.

When Dr. Johan arrived, he was also quick to grasp the seriousness of the situation. The union leaders were called to his office for a meeting—opened, as always during Johan's tenure, with a lengthy prayer from the resident pastor and a Bible reading by Johan. "Behold, how good and how pleasant it is for brethren to dwell together in unity!" he read out, in Telugu, from Psalm 133. Once finished, he slammed the book shut and offered an interpretation of what it meant in the colony. "Here, we're all members of a single family," he said, "This isn't just like a workplace; here we should work together to solve our problems, not start a trade union!"

One of the tailors, in response, set out the union's case: the problems about salaries and job security. Dr. Johan nodded, seemingly in agreement. "But you can't look at what you get as salaries," he said cheerfully. "Think of it as a donation to uplift you a little from your previous standard of living." I squirmed in my chair at the patronizing tone, but resisted the temptation to disagree publicly. Nothing had changed—the court cases did not miraculously disappear and the union did not back down—but at least the doctor had established some ground rules for how these issues would be discussed. His tenure marked a calmer, more civil period in the office.

Unfortunately, it did not last for long. Unhappy with his salary from the start, Dr. Johan soon found a more lucrative posting as a doctor at a private hospital in Sri Lanka. Even before I left the village myself in October 2000, he was gone. By now, there was rising support in the village, and among the Elders, for Das to be reinstated, despite the fact that people seemed to know he owed money to the office. "We've tried these outsiders," the then president explained it to me, "but they don't understand our ways of doing things here. Unless we can get a foreigner—like Emma Cox or you—to come and run things for us, it's better to have someone like Das." Looking at it cynically, having someone who was indebted to the office might also have served the Elders' purposes well: such a leader was likely to yield to their demands.

It was perhaps for this reason that Das seemed less than thrilled at his reappointment as project co-ordinator, but he accepted it. Like almost everything else, he saw it as something that happened to him. Nothing, he told me, had really changed: the court cases still needed to be fought, and colony employees were becoming ever more litigatious.

His attempts to get through to the villagers were not working and, with Dr. Johan's calming influence gone, people were getting vocal about their complaints again. "I brought our advocates here once," Das said, "so I could show them the benefits people received and so they could use this in the labour case. I also wanted them to reason with the villagers. We called a meeting so they could explain the situation to people, but everyone was shouting at the same time, and they were raising all kinds of irrelevant matters. You know what people are like here. One man complained that we hadn't paid to have his legs amputated when he needed them to be, and wanted to know what they were going to do about it! Another stood up and shouted that we hadn't given training opportunities for his son. What had any of this to do with it? The advocates looked around at me and said, 'How long have you worked here? How can you stand this? You'll be driven mad!' I mean, these weren't Daniel's lawyers or the union's—they were *ours*, the Association's. They'd come to explain the situation, but they had to give up and go!"

Despite his efforts, the court cases were becoming more and more farcical. Although they no longer had the vehicle, the President and the Secretary of the Elders and his deputy, Gurumurthy, mostly came along for the ride, trips away from the colony to the court offering a good excuse for special meals and drinking. "If Gurumurthy came along, there would definitely be drinking afterwards," Das said. "He'd demand that we stop on the way back, go to an eating place and send their boy over to the liquor shop to buy some brandy or whisky. He'd drink it on its own, with some ice and some soda; I preferred to drink it with beer."

"I didn't complain because if I'd had a drink at least I could get to sleep, at least for a couple of hours. But then I'd wake up again and lie there worrying. I wasn't drinking continuously like an addict, usually I liked to take only a small quantity. And if the level of worry was very high, well, maybe I would take some more. It's funny, when I used to live on the pavement outside the station, when I had nothing and no-one, I had no interest in drinking or in smoking cigarettes and these kinds of things. It was only because of all these new problems that I developed these habits. I thought, why not? Try it!"

I didn't hear much from Das during the next two or three years, and his account of that period is the least coherent, the least detailed of all those he gave me, despite it being relatively recent. It remained difficult for him to talk about. "The situation became very bad," he said simply. "From 2001, we were attending court every two or three days. There was a lot of time wasted—seven years of going back and forth from the court house—and a lot of money too: nearly Rs400,000 of wasted expenditure."

His relationship with Padma had also lost some of the allure of its earlier days. It was not about escapism any more. "People started to know what was going on and to talk about us," he said. "Some Vijayawada begging people saw us together, and then word got out. She wasn't bothered, but I wasn't happy about it. Someone wrote to members of the management committee about this matter, in 2002 or 2003 I think, I'm not exactly sure when, saying that I wasn't behaving appropriately and shouldn't be in charge. I was sincere in my feelings for Padma, but one thing I didn't like about her was her willingness to talk openly about our affair to people, even here in the village! I'd pass by and she'd come out of her house and say, loudly, 'When are you going to come away with me? Come, and I'll look after you!' So everyone knew, including the Elders. Even her husband must have known, but he never once said anything, never pointed it out. Maybe behind my back he did, but never to my face. Even now he'll come to my house and call me to their house for some special occasion."

"I'd say to Padma, 'How can we just leave? You have a husband, I have a wife and two children. We can't just go!' And she'd get more and more angry about that, complaining all the time that I didn't give her enough support. Things were difficult all around!"

As with most events in his life, change finally came about not as a consequence of his own decision, but on the initiative of others.

Chapter Nine

Moving On

Life in Anandapuram continued to get worse. "I would sit at my desk at work, or lie on my bed in the middle of the night, thinking to myself: 'How can I get out of this job?' Everything was a mess: the committee was taking all these decisions that weren't being followed; no-one was co-operating about the court cases; and I couldn't see any way of paying all my debts." He had tried to resign on several occasions, Das said, but each time the Elders had persuaded him to stay on. They would speak to the committee, they said, get him help with his work.

In the end, though, it was the Elders who paved the way for what he described as his escape, despite the note of regret in his voice when he talked to me about it. "I remember it very well," he told me. "It was February 25, 2005—twenty years to the day that I started working in the office—and a group of Elders came to see me there. They might have spoken first to Emma or the other committee members, I don't know. But they gathered around and the President said to me: 'Das, do you want to resign from your post? If you are not able to do the job any longer, we will accept your resignation.' My immediate feeling was one of relief. 'Now I can finally get out of this job!' I thought. So I told them yes, I was ready to resign, and I got the paper out then and there and wrote my resignation letter. And they said to me that I'd need to pay this and that—the amounts still outstanding as advances; and I'd also need to sign to say that I would take responsibility for various unpaid bills from other people. Someone, for example, had absconded from the village owing the office lots of money. So they put his debts in my name too. There was a builder who I had paid to get official approval of the building work from government inspectors; he had done the work, but he never presented his bills, so that sum was put on my head as well."

"I suppose I shouldn't have signed for these things, but at the time I saw this as an immediate way out from all the pressures. So I thought, okay, I'll write whatever they want me to write, and when the committee meets and calls me to explain myself, then I can explain quite easily. I knew I needed to pay some money—maybe half of it—back to the office, but not all of it, and I felt that it could all be sorted out later on. I wrote the letter and signed it, with the Elders all standing there over me. And then I left, right away. Now at least I could sit in my house without everyone knocking on my door from dawn until midnight, or shouting at me in the streets. I didn't have to put up with people coming to complain about the quality of the food from the kitchen, or the state of the dressing they had got from the clinic. Now I wouldn't need to lie awake worrying about how we would pay the staff their salaries or the rice man's bills."

I have never fully understood why, if he was not responsible for the expenditure outstanding in his name—a sum more than five times his annual salary—he had signed over responsibility for it so easily. If it had been as straightforward as he kept telling me to account for the expenditure, why did he not do so—even now, when I asked him, or, much earlier, in the books? Given his noted skill with numbers, I pressed him, surely he could have found some way of accounting for all this? Das would become visibly distressed during these discussions, banging his forehead with his hands and walking, as well as talking, round and round in small circles. "We will get the books and go through that expenditure line by line if you like," he would say in response to my frustration, "and I can show exactly what was mine and what wasn't. And that's what I can show the committee." But he never did, and the committee never called him to account for himself directly: the evidence, as they saw it, was there in the letter he had signed.

Nevertheless, his immediate emotion on leaving the office was one of relief. The roof of his house was now leaking badly during the monsoon season, requiring him and his family to move their beds around the small room to avoid the water that dripped in through the concrete ceiling or down the walls, but it did not bother him. Now he could sleep through the night. And the size of his debt, to moneylenders and the bank as well as to the office, was so big that it somehow felt beyond his reach: he would never be able to pay everything off whatever he did, so what—as he now seemed to feel—was the point in worrying about it?

My own concern, on hearing at the time that he had finally left the job, was how he and his family were going to survive. Mariya worked part-time, like other village women, in the weaving shed, but she did not make enough money to feed a family, let alone to keep the moneylenders off their backs. Their children were also growing up: Joshua was now ten, and Kaveri was seven. Both of them, Das said, suffered from health problems: ear infections, fevers, stomach upsets—the usual illnesses of childhood in South India, exacerbated by poverty.

His brother Chandra Prakash, who pulled a rickshaw, had somehow saved or borrowed enough money to send his own two sons to a local English medium school, and the contrast between the two sets of cousins was striking. Chandra Prakash's children, when I saw them, were softly spoken and well-groomed; faces always freshly powdered, hair neatly combed and held in place with coconut oil. Their clothes, while not expensive, were always newly laundered and pressed, and they wore rubber flip-flops on their feet. Joshua and Kaveri, by contrast, were unkempt and seldom bothered with footwear. Their clothes were crumpled and full of holes, and—compared to their cousins—their movements were less constrained. People in the village commented on such things: they approved of children who were quiet and well presented, rather than those who ran around wildly and noisily. Such children, people commented sadly, had already been spoiled. Das seemed bemused by them: from his perspective, their behaviours were not a reflection of their upbringing but, more likely, of their mixed caste heritage. The fact that they were half-Madiga was a source of some concern to him but also a kind of explanation for aspects of their characters he did not like or understand. Like their mother, they embodied their caste. "What can we do?" he would ask rhetorically, throwing up his hands in a gesture of despair.

Das was not, in fairness, an entirely distant father, especially compared to some of his peers. Fathers made decisions on behalf of their children, but in many cases left it to the mothers to enforce those decisions. When he was in the village he at least played with and talked to them, affectionately but absent-mindedly tousling their hair as they clambered over him. But, as with other things, he took little direct responsibility for the way they were. Although he did not say so directly, almost everything he did say pointed to a belief that things were simply pre-destined to be a particular way, and there was little that could be done to change them.

Of Joshua's behaviour, he told me: "Really, I am very shocked about how he carries on. I never did any of the things that he does: hunting, fishing, eating fish and mutton. But he not only does all of them, he relishes them! He'll catch small fish by hand when they clear out the fishpond, put them in his pocket and bring them back for his mother to fry. And he uses a catapult to fire at birds and other creatures, like a hunter! I've seen him and his friends go off together with their catapults!"

Kaveri could at least be persuaded to help out in the home: to wash the plates at the hand pump after they had eaten, to sweep the house or to help her mother wash the family's clothes. "But Joshua, he won't do any of these things. When he's eaten his food he just uses the water from his glass to wash the rice from his hand into his plate and he goes away, not even lifting up his plate. I told his mother that she needed to tell him. I even smacked him once or twice, told him that he at least needed to clean his own plate, that this would be a good habit to get into. But Mariya doesn't help. She just says to me, 'Why are you beating him? Leave him be!' So what can I do?"

At the point of Das's resignation from the office Joshua was, at least, attending school most of the time, and Das anyway believed he was sufficiently wily—as he, and before him his own father, had been—to get by whatever happened. "But Kaveri, she's more like her mother, so I worry about her," he said. "I knew she was not going to school and that people were talking about it. It looked bad when even the project co-ordinator's own daughter didn't attend school. But what can we do? She is not going, so she stays in the house. One day the teacher beat her with her stick, so she was not interested to go after that—she was in second class then, I think, so she was about six. She came back home one day at the 10am recess, and never returned. Her books were all there in the classroom, and she said that I would have to collect them: she wouldn't go there alone. We didn't go—we thought we'd leave it for a while and maybe when she forgot about what happened she'd go back. But after about ten days, the teacher finally sent the books back. I think the beating she received on her leg must have really hurt her that time, and nothing would make her return. Even if we sent her in the morning she'd just come back as soon as I went to the office, and I can't keep taking her back. Her mother, she's not educated herself, so she doesn't understand these things. If Kaveri says she doesn't want to go, well, Mariya just thinks, 'Okay then, don't go, you can help me here.' Without my wife's support, there's not much I can do."

Das and I sometimes argued about his fatalistic approach to life. He didn't subscribe intellectually to the doctrine of *karma*—the notion that what happens to us in this life is the consequence of actions in past incarnations. But although people regularly discard the beliefs that once motivated them in response to new evidence or new prejudices, the embodied vestiges of those beliefs are harder to shift. Just as I embodied the Judaeo-Christian notion that people were, as individuals, responsible for their own actions and that actions had direct consequences—however much I recognized those ideas, in the abstract, as distinctive products of Western capitalist thought—so too did Das remain a product of his environment. Like others who considered themselves modern, he rejected *karma* and a belief in fate as the products of superstition and tradition, the kind of thing uneducated villagers believed in. To not believe in them was to set oneself apart. In a world in which so many things really did seem to be out of one's direct control, however, it was hardly surprising that such notions penetrated so deeply. They also offered a good excuse for inaction.

Maybe, I began to think, Das was right to take such an approach to life. While I fretted about what would become of him and wrote to him, pressing him to take control of his situation, to apply for jobs, to find a way to support his family, he stayed at home and waited, apparently passively, for something to happen. "I just sat in the house, wandered around, rested," he recalled of the weeks that followed his forced resignation. "I drank a bit, and—now that I didn't have the office to worry about—I could play cards with people out in the open." Although I found it hard to accept his confidence that all would be okay—or that, even if it was not, there was nothing he could do about it—within a month, things had indeed worked themselves out. Vibulananthan, the director of Tradefair, had sent Das a message asking him if he wanted to come and do some work for the federation. The work was not high level, but it would enable him to feed himself and the family, *and* it took him away from the troubles of Anandapuram and back to Chennai. "Vibulananthan is a good friend," Das said. "He knew me, and he knew what I could do. So he told me that he was happy to find me something to do at Tradefair; I was taken on to look after the store room there at the main office."

After his previous role, it was a welcome relief. He needed to mark orders in and out, package up goods for export, and complete the necessary paperwork. There were no Elders and no angry leprosy patients to answer to. Just his colleagues in the office there, and Vibulananthan, who he would sit and chat with in the evenings, and sometimes help out with his own work. "I slept there in the office itself, in the middle room under the fan. I didn't use the guesthouse room—that didn't feel right—but the floor in the office was cooler anyway, so I was quite comfortable. Vibulananthan would often stay in the office working until beyond midnight anyway, that was his way of working, and so there wasn't time to feel bored or lonely. We'd take tea or coffee together, talk about things in Tradefair and in Anandapuram."

The deal was that he should return to his family in Anandapuram once a fortnight for a weekend, taking the night train back to Chennai on a Sunday evening and being there for work again on Monday morning. Das did not see Padma much during that period, other than to greet her in the street. Neither of them had formally broken off the relationship, but they were in different places, and there was no time. When he was in Chennai he stayed close to the office, talking to the driver and the caretaker of the building, who lived with his wife in a hut at the back of the compound. He also went a couple of times to visit his mother, who was living independently now in a couple of rooms that had been made available to her in another distant relative's house. The relative and his family were away over seas, so it suited them to have someone living on site, and her other needs were met with an allowance from Parvathi's sons. Without Parvathi there to lead conversation, however, meetings with his mother felt awkward. They went through the pleasantries, asked after each other's health and went through the relatives one by one, but beyond that there was not a great deal left to be said. They had spent too many years apart to find common ground now. Das told me that he had mentioned his debts to her at one point, but she had pleaded with him never to ask Parvathi's sons for money. "They have always looked after me, always," she told him. "So please don't ask them for any more. They have done enough."

Das agreed: "All those years Parvathi and her husband and then her children cared for her, much better than her own sons could have done. I am grateful to them for that, they took away that burden from me, so it wouldn't have been right to have asked for help for me."

Instead, his mother would press a token amount of money—a hundred rupees or so—into his palm each time he left and tell him to spend it on the children. She would make him tea and offer him snacks and, if he called near a meal time, she would cook him rice and serve it to him with sambar, rasam, curds and pickles. She would also pass on shirts and trousers that Parvathi's sons had worn and now discarded, often, as Das pointed out to me, for no other reason than that a single button was missing. Judging by the shirts Das's cousins were larger men than he was, and they drooped slightly off his shoulders, but these hand-me-downs meant he did not need to worry about clothes for himself. It was just as well, because there was no spare money around. Vibulananthan paid him a salary of Rs5,000 per month, Rs2,000 of which was sent straight to Mariya, so she could ensure there was food in the house for her and the children to eat. The remaining Rs3,000, according to Das, went on travel, food and out of pocket expenses while he was in Chennai. "There were no cooking facilities in the office, so I had to eat out three times a day. Then there were day-to-day expenses: shaving, soap and shampoo, train tickets back to the village. It was easy to spend everything I was earning."

Most of his meals were taken at the canteen on the corner, a couple of minutes' walk from Tradefair's offices. It was a traditional, Brahmin-run place, and Das liked the food there. The owner sat proprietarily behind a counter at the front on a high chair beneath the fan, quietly taking money from the customers as they left, while the staff—washing up bowls to collect plates in or sponges to wipe over the tables in hand—dashed hurriedly to wherever they were beckoned around the dining room. Downstairs they served tiffins: paper dosas cooked in ghee that were as long as the black marble topped tables, or spongy idlis and deep-fried vadas, all accompanied with sambar and the three chutneys—chilli, mint, and coconut—that made up the colors of the Indian flag. Upstairs, where the mood was more frenetic, lunch and dinner were served in the style it once had been at Das's father's mess: rice, fried vegetable dishes and *papad*, sambar, rasam, curds and lime or mango pickle. They served proper, freshly ground and brewed South Indian coffee downstairs too, presented, as Das liked it, in stainless steel cups with deep saucers in which to pour the coffee back and forth until it reached the right temperature. I had eaten there many times on my visits to Chennai. It was not the kind of place frequented by a metropolitan elite, but neither was it was a poor man's eatery or a student-style mess. Most of the clientele were lower middle class—office clerks grabbing breakfast on the way to work or taking lunch. Das could, I sometimes suggested, have found somewhere cheaper to eat. "But," he told me, "you can't live like that all the time."

Five months after Das started working in Chennai, I returned to India for another fieldwork trip. This time I came to Hyderabad, the state capital, 350-kilometres west of Anandapuram. I had completed my PhD and had post-doctoral funding to carry out research on living with bodily-differences beyond leprosy, and was planning on working with people with cerebral palsy and sight-impairments. Although I could get by in Telugu, Hyderabad has a large Muslim, Urdu speaking, population. I had taken a course in Hindi which, at conversational level, is close enough to Urdu, but I was not sufficiently proficient to interview people in it or to follow fully everything that was being said around me. By the time I had worked out the grammatical structure of my sentence my interlocutors had usually responded to my questions in English. My sense of direction was also appalling, and, to do the multi-sited fieldwork I planned, it would save a lot of time if I had someone to work with.

I had been wondering, initially, whether to recruit an anthropology or sociology post-graduate student from one of the local Universities: someone who would have both the language skills and a sense of what it was I wanted to understand. Too many people who had wanted to work with me in the past had too firm an idea of what it was I needed to know: if I wanted to know about caste, for example, it was difficult to get across that I wanted to know what people thought about it or how it might impinge on their lives; not, as it was often assumed, an official, "correct" version that only certain people could give me. "You don't want to ask these people what they think," one of my previous applicants for the role—a local chicken farmer with a good command of English—had told me. "They'll get all the facts wrong. But if you tell me what it is you want to know I can find out from reliable sources!" I also needed someone who felt at home talking to anyone, whether it was someone begging in the streets or a hospital consultant who would serve as a gatekeeper to accessing people I might work with more closely. In a context where status mattered, this was not as easy as it sounded. I had friends who would have cowered at the sight of a senior administrator, and others who would have squirmed at having to translate my impertinent questions.

In the past, Das had been too busy with his work as project co-ordinator to be my research assistant. Besides, he had been far too embroiled in community affairs to play the role effectively. He had been a major informant though, spending a lot of time chatting to me on my verandah in the evenings, offering important insights on the observations I had recorded that day.

Like me he was interested in reflecting on what people said and did, and seemed to have an instinctive understanding—because rather than in spite of, I fancy, his lack of formal post-school education—of the kind of things I was interested in. Sometime in the period between Das leaving his job in Anandapuram and me arriving in Hyderabad it dawned on me that, if he was not tied to Tradefair, he would make an ideal research assistant. He was fluent in Telugu, Hindu and English, as well as in Tamil and Marathi, should we need them. He could type, of a fashion, and he was happy to mix with anyone, from the likes of Mr. Klausman to the people he had once lived with on the station. I also knew him well, liked him and his company, and I knew that we could work comfortably together. Vibulananthan was supportive of the idea, too, and said he would be happy to consider taking Das back if there was still work for him to do when I returned, a year later, to the UK. "There's a high turnover of staff there," Das told me. "Lots of people don't adjust well to Vibulananthan's way of working: he keeps long hours, expects staff to stay on late into the night if he's there, and wants things done a certain way. I don't mind that, but he knew other people wouldn't stay for so long, so he could be sure there would be a place left for me."

In September 2005, then, Das came to meet me, my partner and my three-year-old son, on the platform at Hyderabad station as we arrived from Delhi. He looked older than the last time I had seen him—his temples were a little greyer and his face more lined—but he looked well and not visibly diminished by all the difficulties I had been hearing about. I was pleased to see him, and grateful for his help in loading my family's luggage for the year from the train and into the taxi he had lined up. Even his experience as a station porter was going to be useful.

The temperature in Delhi, where we had visited friends on the way into the country, had been searing: it was still in the forties despite this being September, and the air was so humid that even walking along the street felt as laborious as wading through wet mud. Here, in Hyderabad, it had clearly been raining and, despite the pollution, after Delhi it felt fresh and relatively cool. Just as I had been when I had arrived in Anandapuram for a prolonged stay six years earlier, I was excited at the prospect of starting new fieldwork.

My intention, at the outset, was that Das would find lodgings somewhere nearby and that we would meet to work each morning. I only had funding for a part-time assistant, so the idea was that he would spend two weeks or thereabouts in Hyderabad, and the rest of the month back with his family in Anandapuram, maybe also finding some temporary work there or back at Tradefair. Das, however, was adamant that it would be pointless paying out money to live somewhere else, and that he would stay with us at the flat I had found and rented out in Abids: it had two bedrooms, so he was happy either to take one of those or to sleep on the floor somewhere in the main living room. If we had visitors he would sleep outside on the large, enclosed balcony. I was, to start with, a little dubious about whether this arrangement would work out. We lived differently to Das and had our own way of doing things. I knew from past experience that he was also particular about the kinds of food he would eat and the context in which he would eat them. I also knew he would disapprove of my occasional practice, when wanting to escape the world of my informants, of going to drink coffee in shopping mall cafes that, although half of the price of a coffee in an equivalent place in the UK, cost thirty times more than they did at a stand in the street. He would also, I judged, be aghast at how much we would sometimes spend on lunch at one of the city's five star hotels (even if he had spent much more in a single day at the race track). Again, by European standards these meals were cheap—twenty-five pounds sterling for the entire family, and two or three hours relishing the cool of the air-conditioning and the comfort of padded chairs without being approached by hawkers or beggars. Even on a UK lecturer's salary it seemed like a bargain. But in Hyderabad it was the equivalent to a maid's monthly salary, and taking Das to such places felt uncomfortable and took away the pleasure. Once, after spending the morning at the height of summer in the hot, basement consulting room of a local doctor and walking some distance in the sun to try to catch a bus to our next location, I had suggested we take refuge in the air-conditioned coffee shop of a three star hotel alongside the bus stop. We were tired, thirsty and hungry, and I thought we could take food there too. Once inside, however, Das—after complaining that "this is the kind of place people come to spend money like water!"—refused to take anything but tea (at Rs60!) on the basis that there was nothing to eat. Nothing on the continental style menu, mainly pizzas and pasta dishes, included rice, and although most of the options contained no meat, Das was not convinced they counted as vegetarian.[1] We ended up taking our lunch at a stand-up tiffin shop next door, batting away the flies as we crammed down our vadas and dosas, both of us in sour moods.

These concerns aside, however, living in the house together worked reasonably well, particularly as I got time together with my family in the weeks when he was back in Anandapuram. The flat came with its own maid, Fatima, who arrived most days to cook, wash the clothes and clean the house, so initially he was also invaluable in navigating the uncharted territory of negotiating our mutual expectations. My feeling, based on my experiences at middle class informants' houses, was that families who could afford maids tended to treat them badly: they worked long hours for low wages and spoke to (or shouted at) them rudely. As I came to understand, however, maids also had expectations of their employers that went beyond what I had seen as a relatively straightforward commercial exchange. The same middle class women who yelled at their servants for not washing the kitchen floor properly or for putting too much salt in the curry were, at the same time, expected to put up loans for medical treatment or to offer a shoulder to cry on when errant husbands squandered their wives' paltry salaries on arrack. In short, the ground rules were different, more feudal, and although I never adjusted to them entirely—I am not enough of a cultural relativist to think it is ever acceptable to beat one's staff—Das was a useful guide on what was and what was not reasonable. He also helped negotiate complex arrangements for covering bus fares and the other expenses that made up her wage packet, and to figure out what work she was actually expected to do.

"She was a very good cook and a hard worker," said Das, "and I liked talking to her and sharing our difficulties in life. We visited her house together once, remember? She lived in similar conditions to how we lived in Anandapuram: in a small, one roomed house with a drunken husband and four children to support!" She had confused him at first: she had what we thought was a Muslim name, but wore a kumkum in the centre of her forehead and painted rangoli patterns on her doorstep each morning like a Hindu, and yet she was a Roman Catholic. Christian converts in Anandapuram often dressed in a particular way, without kumkums or flowers in their hair, as a sign of their piety, but for Fatima, who was not a convert but had been born to a Catholic family, such symbols were unnecessary. She simply dressed as her neighbors and others around her, mostly Hindus, also dressed. Fatima, and various combinations of her four young children, soon became as entangled in the day-to-day life of our household as Das was. Her curries, mostly, at our request, were dahl-based vegetarian dishes, but occasionally she made Hyderabadi biryanis or local fish curries, rich with ground cashew nuts and coconut. She made her own dosas, too, served with garlicky peanut chutney, and perfectly round chapattis, puffed up with air on the flame of our gas hob and kept warm in the insulated casserole containers that all our food came served in. It was an enviable set-up.

As well as approving of the domestic arrangements and the food, Das also enjoyed the work. Our constant movements across the city satisfied his desire never to stay still, and he enjoyed working with a range of people. "Every day we'd be somewhere else, talking to people who were affected by some kind of disability or who worked with them, so it was interesting," he said, recounting it for me several years after the event. "We visited people's houses—where they would bring us tea and coffee and different kinds of snacks, sometimes even meals—and we'd spend time in hospitals, schools, and sitting talking with disabled people who went begging on the edge of the roadside. It was very varied."

We returned, in October that year, to visit Anandapuram for a few days. It was a difficult trip for several reasons. I had not been to the village for a few years—a longer gap than between my usual visits—and there was an exhausting number of people who queued up to see me with requests for help from the charity I was still involved with. The weather was stormy: it was humid and wet, and from dusk until dawn the air was thick with mosquitoes.

The thunder offered a suitable backdrop to the mood, however, because it was during our time in the village that news came of Das's father, who had been away begging in Mumbai. We were sitting outside on the verandah of the Mahila Mandal building at the time, drinking tea, when a girl arrived to say that Sharadha, an old village women who was also in Mumbai, had called the public phone in the village centre and needed to speak urgently to Das or his brother, Chandra Prakash. Something had happened, the girl said, to Das's father. Das rushed off to the pay phone and waited for Sharadha to call back again. Timothy, it transpired, was dead. After putting the phone down and returning in silence to the verandah, I saw Das cry for the first time: not the wailing and head-beating that was the common response to a death, but slow, quiet sobs, his body gently convulsing. I patted him uneasily on the back.

Timothy, he told me, had not been well for some time. But his wife, Elizabeth Rani, had insisted that he continued to go begging, despite exhortations from him and his brother that he should stay in the colony. "They were both on the custodial care scheme," said Das, "so they had a small income coming in and could have got by, but Elizabeth Rani, she always wants more: gold ornaments, new saris. And if he stayed here in the house she used to go on at him, make more and more demands, so I think he found it easier to stay in Mumbai." Timothy was, in any case, eighty years old, so his death—ten years after he almost died the first time, just before Joshua was born—was not in itself a shock. What saddened Das and his brother in particular was that he had died begging on the streets. It took a while for the news to filter through: Sharadha was not the most coherent of witnesses. A former teashop owner, she was now very elderly herself, and was seldom sober. When her story was finally corroborated, it transpired that Timothy's fellow leprosy sufferers had found him too far away from the begging camp to carry him back there. Even if they could have done, there was no way they could get him on a train for the 24-hour journey back to Anandapuram. He had probably already been dead for several hours. In the end, they left him there, his body pushed to the side of the road, for the municipality to collect when they cleaned the streets the next morning.

"We'd planned to go back to Hyderabad the next day, October 28, but we put the trip off while my brother and I talked about what to do, whether we needed to go to Mumbai," Das remembered. "Charles Wesley's daughter Annamma and her uncle, Ramdas, did though—she was training to be a nurse in one of the big Hyderabad hospitals. They were on the Delta Passenger to Secunderbad and it crashed, killing hundreds, including those two. If my father hadn't died, we would have been on that train. So Joshua saved him ten years ago; this time he saved us, by dying!" He let out a hollow laugh in recognition of the dark absurdity of it all.

Back in Hyderabad, as time went on we fell into a rough pattern. Nearly every evening we would turn up for an outpatients' clinic at a large hospital run by a neurosurgeon for children with cerebral palsy, where we would spend time first in the cavernous waiting room, chatting, when we could, with families waiting to see the doctor. Dr. Sharma would call us in once he had a patient he thought we might be interested in. Privacy was much less of an issue in consulting rooms than it seemed to be in the West: the doctor would happily be describing the operation a patient needed to have or examining an x-ray as the next patient and her family were led into the room by his peon, Das and I present throughout. He spoke to us between patients, or called another of his peons to bring us tea, coffee, or a variety of different snacks. "You must try the small samosas they sell over the road!" he would say one day, calling for his assistant and giving him some money to buy the required snack. Or: "I saw some new sweetmeat in the store on the corner when I went past this morning. Venkata Rao! Come, you need to go and buy some sweets for these fellows!"

He also found us a room, adjacent to his own, where we could sit and talk to the patients before and after he had seen them, sometimes making plans to visit them in their homes. Das liked Dr. Sharma and his company, asking him questions of his own and offering opinions on patients and other matters as well as discussing the research. Dr. Sharma never seemed to mind, and—a northern Indian without a good grasp of Telugu—he often used Das as an interpreter when the patients did not speak English. Only once in all the time we were visiting him did I notice his eyes fall momentarily onto Das's shirt cuff, well-frayed and done up with a safety-pin. Das was difficult to place socially: confident and polite without showing the deference in words or manner that might betray lowly origins, he was also quick to drop into conversation that he was a Tamil Brahmin and had managed an NGO. Yet he wore dusty, scuffed sandals that had been repaired many times; not-quite-fitting but good quality shirts that were past their best and never tucked in, and was equally at ease with the peons who led in the patients and delivered our snacks.

Likewise, he got on well with the people we met in a disabled colony on the northern peripheries of the city: a mixed group of Hindus, Muslims and Christians who relied mainly on rag-picking and begging to sustain themselves. The government had allocated them the land, but beyond that they had very little external support, and were used to living on their wits. One woman died by dousing herself with kerosene and setting herself alight during an argument in the period we were visiting, and her death scarcely raised a batted eyelid. This was a village where, when communal rioting had spread through the old city a few years earlier, neighbours in the colony had burned down one another's houses, only to find themselves, in the aftermath, still living next door to the same people. They were poor—so poor that many of the children had the chestnut colored hair associated with malnutrition—and they were hardened. Anandapuram seemed like a middle class enclave by comparison. But Das didn't baulk at them and their often foul language, even if took some persuading to get him to translate threats to rub vaginas with chillies or to engage in anal sex with someone's grandmother. He sat alongside them on his haunches on the ground, chatting, laughing, joining in the banter, and asking them the questions I wanted him to ask. Within a bus ride of these trips, however, he could be sitting in a government office or across the table from the gatekeeper of a disability NGO who would be demanding to know the hypothesis we were trying to test with our research. We were both enjoying ourselves.

We also paid weekly visits to an eye hospital, where we were given free run of the waiting room in the rehabilitation centre, and access to the patient canteen, where we took our lunches. The waiting room was long and narrow, brightly lit with tube lights and lined on either side with wicker armchairs. There was a television on the wall in one corner and, if there was a major cricket match on, there was no chance of getting Das to talk about anything else to the patients, most of whom—along with the medical staff—would likewise be transfixed by the screen. Patients came from all over Andhra and sometimes from further afield, including a man from Mumbai and an elderly woman from Rajasthan. As many of them had long waits before or between appointments, there was usually plenty of time for them to talk to us. "Just do it for 'time pass'" Das would tell those who expressed initial reluctance. "Why unnecessarily sit here getting bored when you could be speaking to us?"

Through those encounters we also worked our way into the homes of some of those we met, visiting them for less formal conversations about their experiences of living with impairments and, many times, to share tea or coffee and sometimes food. If we managed to visit several households in one go Das would often complain, jokingly, as we were thrown from side-to-side on the bumpy bus ride home, that his stomach was awash with tea and Britannia milk biscuits: refusal felt impolite, so we always accepted what we were offered.

One of the things we noticed about the eye hospital was its unpredictability. Some days there would be patients coming in and out from the time we arrived until the time we left, with us interviewing as many as twenty patients and having more to visit later on. There were other days on which we did not encounter a single patient. Although those occasions were initially frustrating, they also offered good opportunities for us to talk through, uninterrupted, the work we had already done and, less formally, to chat about our own lives. I had not planned by then to write Das's biography, but going back through my notes on our conversations from that period helped form many of the subsequent questions I put to him.

It was there, in that waiting room, that Das first talked, at length, about his relationship with Padma, about his own marriage, and about the problems that had precipitated his demise in Anandapuram. In respect of the latter, the conversations were often unsatisfactory, Das repeating again and again that the enormous debts he accrued, in the office and among moneylenders, were mainly to do with high interest rates and unaccounted for expenditure that had wrongly been attributed to him by the Elders when he resigned. I knew little, at this stage, of his penchant for gambling, even though later, when I did, he denied he ever made heavy losses that way. Passing the time, we would try to list his debts in my notebook, recording alongside them the monthly interest rates that were being charged, who he owed them to, and how best to start paying them back.

"So this woman here," I'd say, jabbing at a name with the tip of my pencil, "is charging you 5 percent per month on what's now a debt of Rs10,000. So how about you pay her, say, Rs1,500 a month . . ."

"Yes, but she is not pressing me so much for money at the moment, I think it's better that I pay some of this man's dues—just a couple of thousand—to keep him quiet, and then I go back to back to her in a few months," he would reply, pointing out another name on the list.

"But he's only charging 3 percent, so surely it makes more sense to pay her off first, then . . ."

"Don't worry about her, I can try to convince her to accept less interest, but the others I need to pay first, especially those who are asking me all the time for money. And the office, well, that can wait, and later I can explain to the management committee about how most of that shouldn't be in my name anyway."

And so on. We would go over and over the figures, trying to match up his income to a credible plan for paying off the debt. Although it felt like a game, sitting there alone in the relative comfort of the eye hospital waiting room, playing around with figures, the reality was depressing. Even if we excluded all the money he owed to the office and he continued to earn as he was, there was no realistic chance of him paying everything off before he reached sixty, the official retirement age, in five years' time. Perhaps that was why he had given up on my suggestion to pay off the most expensive debts first, before focusing on the remainder: whichever way he approached the problem, there was no obvious solution.

The list, as it turned out, was also woefully incomplete. Despite assurances that he had remembered everyone to whom he owed money, on several occasions later on he asked me for advances to pay debts to people he had not yet mentioned. "The best thing," he said to me one evening back in the kitchen of the flat, having psyched himself up to approach me, "would be if you could give me an advance of Rs10,000 on my salary. Then you can cut Rs2,000 for the next five months. That way I can pay off this lender, who is now going to my house and pressing my wife for the money, in one lump sum. That will stop the interest also." He talked in hushed tones, head down to avoid eye contact. I hated these conversations as much as he did.

In the end, I conceded, although I was concerned that he would not have enough money left from his Rs8,000 salary to pay other debts and support his family adequately. I was also worried that he might spend the money before he got to the moneylender. When he came to me after three months and said that, now his earlier debt was almost paid back, could I advance him Rs20,000, I said no: for one thing, there were not enough months remaining for the outstanding sum to be repaid unless I cut practically his entire salary, and although he was unperturbed by this, I was concerned there would be insufficient money left for his family.

"That's not a problem," he said, "Mariya's paid most of what we owed the rice man, so we can get more credit from him again now."

"But what's the point," I said, "in trying to pay all these debts off if you're just going to rack up new debts to replace them again?"

The inequalities between us, disguised most of the time as we lived and worked together, made me feel awkward. I knew more about Das's personal finances than I did about any of my friends or family back in the UK, and I would never have ventured to interfere so forensically in how they might manage their debts. At the same time, though, I did have more of a vested interest in Das's financial position: as well as having brokered the original loan that was supposed to give him a clean start back in 1996, I had also given him a larger sum in 2001, with the same purpose in mind. His debts had been keeping me awake at night and, at the time, I happened to have £2,000 in my bank account. What was the point in having money sitting there, I had reasoned, when a friend badly needed it. Making him less dependent on village moneylenders, I had also thought, would make him less vulnerable as project co-ordinator: more able to stand up to the Elders and anyone else without fear of reprisals. After prolonged discussions by email—precursors to the notes and plans we drew up between patients in the eye hospital—I eventually sent him a check. I was not entirely convinced that I was doing the right thing, but after weeks of posing endless questions about moneylenders and their respective rates, to have said no at that stage would have felt immoral; a reinforcement of the power differentials between a white westerner and an impoverished Indian that I so much wanted to avoid.

At the time I had asked Das to let me know as soon as it felt things were slipping out of control again, and he promised me he would. The trouble was, at that stage his moneylenders were putting so much pressure on him to pay them something that he would probably have agreed to anything. In the event, although Das continued to write to me, and acknowledged receipt of the check, he did not mention his finances again, and neither did I push him.

It was only during his final weeks in the office, when word got out about how much Das owed in advances, that I realized he was in trouble again.

"How is it," I asked him in the auto rickshaw back home from the hospital one evening, "that you got into so much debt after having the whole lot cleared only a couple of years before? I understand about the office money— I can see the logic of that—but what about your personal debts to money-lenders? You were earning a salary still, why couldn't you live off that?"

Das laughed. "When I first married and lived in the colony, I earned less than Rs1,500 a month and we managed. I had no habits, no drinking or anything, and somehow it was enough. But the bigger my job got, the higher the salary, the more I spent and the more stressed I got. It would have been better to stay at the lower salary I think . . ."

"Yes, yes," I snapped back irritably. It had been a long day and we had been talking about money for several hours already. "But you're still not answering my question. If you had a clean slate in 2001, and if you've never lost any money gambling or spent anything on Padma, where does all that extra money go?"

"Like I said, the court cases . . . the coming and going. It swallowed up everything: money I took in advances, but my salary too. Yes, I made some mistakes. I didn't account for things properly. And of course there were some debts remaining that we hadn't paid by then."

"But why not?!" I pushed him on his last point. Usually I would have given up. "We made a list, remember, of *everything* you owed—you promised me that it was everything—and I gave you enough to pay all of them back, so why were there still debts outstanding?"

"Tut!" Das was becoming jittery, and the auto driver—alerted by the sound of our rising voices—was looking at us in his mirror. "We paid off all those that were urgent, all those that needed to be paid. But some of them weren't pressing and could wait longer. Some of them we could pay some amount to and they were satisfied, so where was the urgency to pay them everything?"

"Because I gave you the money *specifically* to pay *everyone*!" I was shouting now, and my heart was beating fast. This was a discussion we had been hedging around for months. "That's what we agreed!"

"There were some other expenses we had in the house that we needed to cover," said Das, his voice also rising. He waved his hands dismissively in the air, as though I was losing the main point in the details. "Clothes for the family, repairs to the building, the new covered verandah . . ."

"The new verandah! You paid for that *new* verandah, with the money I gave you to clear your debts!?" I was staring right at him, incredulous.

"Pah! It's started to fall down already!" he responded bitterly, as if, I suppose, to suggest that the verandah was a side issue. Many of his neighbors, after all, had far grander enclosed verandahs than this one. But it had eaten up more than a third of the money I had given him.

"Okay, okay, I'm sorry, what can I tell you?" said Das, finally, shrugging his shoulders defeatedly, trying to calm me down. The auto had already parked up in the bazaar near to our flat so we could get down and buy bananas before walking the rest of the way home. The driver had turned around in his seat and was watching us, intrigued, and in no hurry for us to get down. We continued our argument—in circular vein—as we walked back, Das trying to keep far enough ahead to avoid face-to-face confrontation, me raising my voice above the furore of the market so he could still hear.

This, and a similar quarrel we had while crossing the road at a major intersection one morning, nearly getting ourselves run over by a bus in the process, was the most heated of our arguments during the time we worked together that year. Das was less specific in his recollection of them—or at least in recounting them to me. "We had some arguments and differences of opinion about my style of living and my work as the project co-ordinator," he said, laughing sheepishly, when he got to this point in his story during our later interviews. Pressed to elaborate, he shrugged his shoulders. "We just argued, that's all. At the time, you advised me to more careful with how I spent my money. Just eat rice and dhal for Rs8, you told me, then you'll be able to start clearing your debts, but what you don't understand is that it's very difficult to live like that all the time. And we had a few differences on some other things, but mostly the experience was good. There were lots of new friends, new interesting people to speak to."

Despite the intensity of our some of our arguments, however—or perhaps it was a consequence of them—there was one final financial transaction with Das that went beyond his salary repayments that year. One afternoon—again in the eye hospital—he took an official letter out of his pocket to show me. Judging by the number of creases there were in the paper it had been read and re-folded many times, and I was aware that he had been unusually distracted for the past few days. I took it and read it. The letter was from the State Bank of India, from which Das had apparently taken a loan for a sum, with interest, now worth Rs30,000. As he had only made one or two payments before defaulting on the loan and had ignored previous requests for repayments, unless he took immediate action the bank was going to reclaim his house, which he had put up for security.

I didn't respond immediately. I was now passed getting angry about debts that Das had failed to mention in our previous conversations. Anyway, this one did not seem to count, Das implied, because it was from the bank and not a moneylender. But I also foresaw a way of ending our painful discussions about his debts. I would, I told him a few days later, pay off the bank in order to save his home for his family, but that would be it: I would continue to pay him his salary for the few months still remaining, but I would not give him further advances, loans or handouts, and he was not to ask for them again. I realized, of course, that it would not necessarily stop him from doing so, but at least I would have a readymade answer. In addition, I would travel back to Anandapuram with him to go to the bank and pay in the money in person: I wanted to be sure this time that the whole sum was cleared. Even then, he tried to convince me, as we travelled back on the train, that it might be better to pay just some of the loan, enough to satisfy the bank and prevent them from claiming his house. "Then," he said hopefully, "I could use the rest of the money to pay off some of the other money lenders."

"This is the deal," I growled back. "I pay it all, in one lump sum, and it's over. Otherwise nothing."

I worried, too, about what would become of Das and his family when the work with me was over in September 2006. As the time got closer, I helped him to put together a CV, and spent hours going through the small ads in the newspaper, circling jobs I thought he could do. Das was dubious. "Who's going to want a fifty-six-year-old man, a cured leprosy patient?" he said. "I haven't got a degree or anything, only a school leaving certificate, and I'm not the kind of person to get the kinds of jobs they advertise in the papers." He also seemed confident that, once all the fuss about his debts to the office had blown over, he would probably be reinstated again as project co-ordinator: a prospect I thought as unlikely as it was possible to be, given that no progress had been made in resolving his outstanding dues, and that a new outsider had already been appointed in his place. Anyway, I was determined to prove him wrong about his unemployability elsewhere, and got him to ring up one of the numbers about a job as an office assistant in a small, private company. He conceded to go along with me for an interview, but when we got there they told him, apologetically, that the vacancy had already been filled, earlier that day. "What did I tell you?" he said. There were clearly things that I was not going to change. I decided to step back from trying to micro-manage Das's affairs.

Although I stayed on in Hyderabad after Das left in September until the end of the year, I did not see him again until I returned to Anandapuram for six weeks in the summer of 2008, to conduct some research—again with him as my assistant—on youth suicide. The first month after he left I was knocked out with typhoid and dengue fever; when I next went to the village, to say farewells before returning to the UK for Christmas, Das had already left for Chennai. He was, his wife told me, back working with Vibulananthan at Tradefair. Once again, he seemed to have landed on his feet.

NOTE

1. For a nuancing of the veg: non-veg split, see Staples, "Go on, just try some!"

Chapter Ten

The Wheel Keeps Turning

Within two months of leaving Hyderabad, Das was comfortably ensconced in one of the VIP guest bedrooms at a smart new training complex, 20 miles out of Chennai. He was there because Tradefair's boss Vibulananthan, on hearing that Das was free, had found him another job, this time caretaking the facility when it was hired out for training programmes. He liked the work. "I didn't have to cook or clean up for them," he told me, "but I did have to distribute the provisions to those working in the kitchen and mark them out in the stock records, and receive the guests—trainees from government departments and other places—when they arrived, make sure everything was working for them." He ate food from the kitchen along with the workshop delegates, who slept in purpose-built dormitories. The centre was in a relatively remote campus, surrounded by woodland, so there were few other distractions for him to spend his earnings on.

He would have been happy enough to stay there longer, despite the sense of isolation between delegations of trainees, but there were other things for him to do back at HQ. Tradefair had opened a showroom in a salubrious Chennai suburb, where it displayed and sold craftwork produced by the federation's member groups, Anandapuram's weavers and tailors among them. The intention was to break into the new middle class domestic markets that were springing up, and it was a smart shop, pleasantly scented with incense and kitted out with dark-wood panelling and carefully back-lit shelving units.[1] Sales, so far, were not high, but it was also seen as a place to take buyers to that would give them a better feel for how the products might appear in their own outlets elsewhere.

"Vibulananthan wanted me there to check through all the sales statements and to bring the books up to date, check the daily cash books and that sort of thing, so I was mostly in the office at the back," Das said. "If foreigners came in though, I'd often be called out to speak to them because I knew English better than the other staff." From his days as a hotel tout and tourist guide he also knew how to turn on the sales patter, and he enjoyed encounters with new people.

Das spent around two months in Tradefair's showroom, on and off, travelling there with the other staff from the federation's headquarters in the jeep unless Vibulananthan had other tasks he needed him for. "There were more staff at HQ by then too," Das said, "and the guest room had now been turned into an office. It wasn't possible for me to stay there overnight any more, so I found a room in Villivakkam. It was a simple place: there were no cooking facilities, and I shared a common bathroom, but it was all right, and it only cost Rs600 a month."

There was not much time for anything else beyond work. "In the evenings, when I went to my place, maybe it would already be 8:30pm, so I'd just have a bath, wash my clothes, and then I'd simply lie on the bed in my vest and lunghi for a while and read—just a Tamil detective novel or something I'd have picked up from the station or a bookstand. Then in the mornings I'd be up at around 6 or 6:30am, and would wash, clean my teeth, go for breakfast, then go directly to Tradefair.

"For food, at lunchtime I'd eat a packet meal from nearby the office: just curd or *sambar* rice, something simple like that, in one of the tea shops. I didn't bother with full meals, most of the time, and I only ate at cheap hotels. In the evenings, I'd get something on the way back to room, but it would be tiffin items—I only took food [ie rice] once, and even then not full meals. At my age, you don't need so much. And in Chennai you can get good food from tea stalls: tamarind rice, lemon rice, sambar rice, maybe a *vada* or two. That's enough. And then in the evenings, it was always tiffins. I very much like tiffins. Sometimes I'd have *puri*s with potato curry, or sometimes *brinji*—you'd like it, it's a kind of special vegetable mixed rice you only get in Tamil Nadu. It's different to *pulao*, easier to digest, and it contains vegetables like carrots, peas and beans, with a little chilli, salt and, of course, rice. There's some masala there too. I often had that in the evenings." Despite having little money—and despite having adjusted his diet to meet his income—it was still possible to eat very well in South India if you knew where to look. Judging by Das's descriptions—and, for that matter, by the food we ate when we were together—he always managed to feed himself properly when he was away from home, even if a meal without copious mounds of rice was not really considered eating at all.

Other than the quality of the food, however, the new lifestyle held few other attractions. "It was okay," he said, "but it was a machine-like routine, and I got fed up with it sometimes, just going and coming. I was especially fed up with the bus. Often I couldn't get on the first three or four that came because of the heavy rush. So although it was only 10km from where I was staying to the office it would take me an hour and a quarter to get there, because I needed to change buses. And once I got to Tradefair, if they wanted me in the showroom I'd need to go off again with the other staff in the jeep. In the evenings I'd go from wherever I was directly to the room."

There was no time, he told me, for anything other than work, but he did have Sundays off, and he would use that time to go to the cinema, to hang out at the central station—where he still knew, to greet, many of the porters and hawkers who lived there—or, as he did a couple of times, visit his mother. He claimed to have avoided the race track most of the time he was there, although he did admit, when I pushed him, to going "maybe once or twice, when it was very boring, on a Sunday, if I needed a change or if I wasn't going back to the colony. But it was very rare. I got Rs2,000 taken out my salary and sent home already, and by the time my feeding costs and my rent had been taken out there wasn't much left to gamble with."

It is true that the time available for going to the races was limited. In theory, he was supposed to return home once a fortnight to see his family, as he had done previously when he worked in Chennai. As had happened toward the end of his time in Hyderabad, however, he did not always arrive back at work as expected on Monday mornings. In Hyderabad, he would call—often a day or two later—to say that his wife or one of the children had been sick and that he had needed to take them to the doctor. On other occasions he said his wife had simply made a fuss about him leaving her again and persuaded him to stay back another night. It was frustrating, especially if we had made appointments, but not especially remarkable in the context of how people in Anandapuram had always worked. He never complained, after all, about being dragged backwards and forwards across the city to meet informants until late in the evening, and was happy to stay up discussing our research late into the night if the need arose. His absences, though, were becoming more regular. Vibulananthan, when I bumped into him at a meeting a year or so later, reported similar experiences in Chennai. It may have been that, as a man in his late 50s who had drunk too heavily for too long Das now found the journeys exhausting, particularly as worries about his debts were keeping him awake at night again. But his extended absences were also, I think, because he did not always go home directly to the colony, something I discovered several times when I tried to get in touch with him. Maybe he went to Vijayawada or some other place enroute to drink, gamble or meet up with Padma, although he claims that by now their affair was virtually over. Perhaps he was just trying to avoid his creditors.

Unlike when he was at Ultra Marine Blue all those years before, Das did at least stick out the job, difficult bus rides included, this time around, and, in the end, he was pleased he did. Two years after the tsunami had wrecked the livelihoods of many who lived along India's Coromandel coastline, Tradefair had won a contract to conduct a survey of those who had suffered heavy losses and who might benefit from income generation loans.[2] As with all major disasters, there were beneficiaries as well as losers, and this time Das was, at least for a time, one of the winners. The survey team Vibulananthan had drawn together spoke, for the most part, good English, but many of them were not native to Tamil Nadu, and they needed someone who could translate Tamil into English and Hindi, conduct basic questionnaires, and record the data. Das could do all these things and, with the cashbooks at the showroom now up to date, he was available.

As far as Das was concerned, this was the best of all the jobs he had at Tradefair. "I liked it very much," he said. "We weren't ever tied to one place, there was lots of travelling here and there, meeting new people all the time, and the work itself was interesting. And because we were away from HQ, sleeping at a centre from which we were driven out to the survey villages each morning, there were no costs either: no food expenses, no travel—everything was taken care of!"

They worked with communities around Pondicherry, Cuddalore and Marakkanam, along with teams of volunteers from local colleges. "We'd have an address of a village, and we'd go there, find the village head, and ask him to call together people who had been affected by the tsunami. Otherwise we'd just go house-to-house, knocking on people's doors or calling out. When we found the right people, I would ask the survey questions and, as I translated the answers, those working with me would make notes."

"We'd tell them why we had visited and ask them what their previous jobs had been, before the tsunami. Most of them had been fishermen, so we'd also ask if them if there were other skills they had, or other ideas for generating income. Sometimes, we'd explain to them, it might be difficult for them to raise enough income from fishing alone, but that we might be able to get them help with training or loans that would help them to do other things, like setting up small shops, for example. It was a case of motivating them."

"The next stage was for people to be selected for the loans on the basis of the information we collected. I wasn't a part of that—it happened sometime later on—so I can't say who got the money or whether they were able to pay it back or not. Some of them just wanted Rs10,000 or so to set up a petty shop from their own house; others wanted to buy fish and sell it at market, or to set up fish drying businesses. Some just wanted money for new fishing nets, or to repair the ones they had. Or they might ask for computer training for their sons and daughters, or for money to buy an auto rickshaw or some buffalo for milk. They asked for a whole range of things. But most of them didn't want to give up fishing—it was their way of life."

As was so often the case, Das remained cynical about the value of the project as a whole. "In the places we visited," he said, "the fishermen often seemed to be in a better position then their neighbours, who didn't fish, but who hadn't been directly hit by the tsunami. Many of them had motor scooters, or children who had jobs or small businesses. It's true that the tsunami might have affected their business a bit, but I'd say that in more than half the cases—say 60 percent—the people we met didn't really *need* rehabilitation or tsunami relief. Their lives hadn't been ruined. That was my observation."

"But this project wasn't about looking at whether the fishermen were rich or poor, or if there were other people who might also be very poor but whose jobs, perhaps because they didn't have any to start with, weren't affected by the disaster. For the purposes of what we were doing, all fishermen were the same. If they had lost a boat, they would be provided with a new one. But the poorest, they were still poor: they didn't know how to approach those giving out the money and make their case. They were just workers, no? People without proper houses, who would be out all the time working for daily wages on construction sites, or carrying things on their backs. And those people, they need money for rice, they can't afford, even if we give them a loan, to invest in the future."

These were, I thought, useful observations, and I was interested to learn how the project organizers responded to them. For Das, however, there had been no formal context in which to share these opinions. "There was some training before," he said, "but after I had done my bit I wasn't involved with how the data was used, and I could only record the information given to me in the form that it was asked for. We weren't asked for additional details, or to give our opinions. It was up to the student volunteers and their professors, who guided them, to come up with their own conclusions, and I wasn't involved with any of that." With large sums of money to be distributed in order for the project to be dubbed successful, I suspect—sharing with Das a cynicism about how such schemes are administered—that such observations would anyway have been unwelcome: beneficiaries who could show tangible outcomes from their loans—the presence of a shop to be photographed, for example—were more satisfactory for donors than the poorer but transient beneficiaries who might eat up the money.[3]

In any case, in the end, Das was not around long enough to see how the project panned out. He would have been happy to have stayed on longer, working, as he had been, for ten days in the field followed by ten days back at HQ or in the showroom, but an event in February 2007 changed all that. It was during one of the periods when Das was back in the office, and he had travelled in to work on the buses as normal. When he arrived, the office peon ran out to greet him in the courtyard. There had been a phone call, he said, from Das's relatives: his mother had been involved in an accident and was dead. It had happened the day before, but by the time word had got through to them and they had called Tradefair, Das had already left for the evening to his room.

His mother was seventy-eight, so Das was not entirely surprised, although he was shocked by the manner in which it had taken place. Subbalakshmi had left the house with two other elderly women, both neighbors, to attend the temple early in the morning. "She lived in a quiet suburb," Das said, "not some busy, city centre kind of place where there was lots of traffic, but one of those mini vans, delivering mineral water containers, came round the corner, too fast, lost control and then ran into the women as they were crossing the road."

"Apparently, my mother saved the other two by pushing them out of the way. One of them was injured and the other one wasn't hurt at all. But my mother took the full impact, and, as she was already quite frail and thin, it hit her hard. She died on the spot, maybe it gave her a heart attack. One of the ladies ran back to the house and informed the people who lived there, and they rushed out straight away and carried her body back, putting it out on the verandah. They immediately called the three brothers, Parvathi's sons, who looked after her: one in Muscat, one in the UK, the other in Abu Dhabi, and all three of them came back to India on the next flight. They were all there that night or early the next morning; I was only a few miles away, but they managed to get there before I did!"

On hearing the news, Das rang Anandapuram to inform his own brother, Chandra Prakash, but they knew it was too late to get him down for the funeral: the train took eight hours or more, and the rites needed to be performed before then. It was agreed that Das would represent them, as her oldest son, and that Chandra Prakash would arrive as soon as he could to help finalize her affairs.

"I rushed off once I'd spoken to my brother and arrived at my mother's house by 11 o'clock. Her body wasn't there by then, it had been taken to the hospital, and she was there with the three sons. I waited and, after half an hour, the ambulance came to return her body, and the three brothers carried her out. We sat there, together, weeping for some time, and then, at around 3pm in the afternoon, we went to the cremation ground. It was a kilometre or so from the house, not far, and we carried her body there."

Das led the procession, carrying the pot with a ghee-flame that, traditionally, is carried by the grandson. "When we got there," he said, "we put her body on the pyre, performed some Hindu rituals, and then we put the firewood on to her body, followed by dung cakes, then some kerosene oil. I took a piece of burning coal and placed it into the pot, which I also put on the fire. Normally you'd break the pot on the back of the dead person's head, but we did it a bit differently. Then the fire spread to her face, I poured on the ghee, and the fire slowly grew very big. Within half an hour everything was finished. We returned to the house and had a bath there." It was a very different send off to that of his father's, a year and a half earlier, in Mumbai.

Chandra Prakash arrived the next morning, and the pair of them met the three brothers at what had been Subbalakshmi's room. "They showed us everything that had belonged to our mother, including all her bank books and everything, and handed over the work of distributing her things and closing up the place to their sister's husband. The couple were still living in Chennai, so they could deal with all that. One of his relatives had a transport company, so everything was packed up and taken away in one of their vehicles the next morning, and they wrote us checks for all the money she had left."

"They had been her guardians, responsible for looking after her, but they gave everything to us," Das said, still slightly awed at their generosity. "My mother left around Rs3 lakhs— Rs150,000 each—and seven or eight thousand rupees in cash in the house, as well as a few gold ornaments. They handed over everything. They also said that there was some money deposited in our children's names, which would mature in a few years' time. They would have Rs100,000 each."

It looked as though Das had been saved again. Parvathi's sons did not stay long: once they had administered Subbalakshmi's funeral and put her affairs in order, they flew back to their respective countries. Das decided not to stay at Tradefair after that. "Each time I saw her, my mother had told me that I shouldn't be there, that I should be at home with my family," he said. "I kept telling her that I would be, soon, and now that she was gone I felt I had to honour her wishes." Vibulananthan did not try to stop him.

It took thirty days for the checks the brothers had given them to be cashed and, once his half of the money was in his account, Das said he distributed it to those he owed. "It didn't cover everything, and within a day the whole lot was gone!" he said, but it very clearly brought him a peace of mind he had not experienced for a long time. His mother died in February 2007, and the difference in him was still noticeable when I visited Anandapuram in July that year, to undertake more research, again with Das as my assistant, on suicide among young people in the village. His hair was grayer than when I had last seen him—although that might have been because he was due for one of his hair-does—but he was calmer, happy to be back in the village, untroubled now by moneylenders and banks demanding cash. The house looked much the same: rain still leaked down into the main room, and the painted walls were even grimier than when I had last seen then, but his mother's sofa now took pride of place down one wall, and an electric cooler, which they used only as a fan, took up almost a quarter of the space.

Mariya's mood, too, was visibly brighter. Every time I went to the house that summer she proudly served me tea in a small china cup with a daffodil painted on the side—one from Subbalakshmi's modest collection. She had also acquired a batch of new sarees, and a small solid gold Ganesh ornament that she wore on a gold chain around her neck. "Don't let Das pawn it!" I joked, and she said he would have to cut her throat first.

It was also the first time Das had ever asked me to dinner in his house. Elizabeth Rani, his widowed step-mother, often brought me filter coffee in the mornings, and he had sometimes commissioned his brother to prepare

Tamil specialities and to serve them to us at his house but, despite having eaten all around the village—I had even been served dhal and fried greens on the streets when I visited those begging in Mumbai— I had never dined in his own place. Mariya's cooking, he had always said, was not suitable for inflicting on guests.

In the event, however, the meal was delicious. Mariya cooked, hunched in the small kitchen at the front of the house over a kerosene stove, and Das flapped around her, instructing her to add more salt or chilli powder, or directing which serving vessels the various dishes needed to be set out in. There was another visitor in the village who knew Das that day, a representative from the Bangalore NGO Emma Cox now worked for, so he was also invited, and we sat next to each other on the floor, our backs against the sofa, steel plates placed on reed mats before us, incense sticks burning all around. First there was lemon rice, dotted with nuts and mustard seeds, chilli-coated potato crisps and milk sweets, bought in from the bazaar; then white rice, along with individual bowls, which Das or Mariya served us from, of fried ladies' fingers, potato curry and dhal, followed by sambar, rasam, curds and pickle. Das talked us through each dish, enquiring at each stage along the way whether everything was all right: enough salt? Enough chilli? I had to lie on the sofa afterwards, replete, while Mariya brewed more tea. Those months were the happiest I had ever seen her.

Without any income other than the few hundred rupees Mariya brought in as a member of the custodial care scheme funded by Mr. Klausman, I was concerned that it would not last. Das claimed he went to Vijayawada to seek work—"where I might have met up briefly with Padma, but there wasn't a lot between us by then"—but mostly he enjoyed the sense of relief that his problems were in abeyance, spending his time playing carrom board or cards and taking trips out to the local cinemas. In September, he joined Mariya on the custodial care program, a scheme intended to provide two hours of light duties a day to those who were not fit enough for begging or full-time work, but not ready yet to join the feeding list, which just provided them with meals, clothes and washing materials. I am not sure that either Mariya or Das were the kind of candidates originally envisaged as beneficiaries of the program, but Mariya—who was genuinely physically weak and had difficulty in keeping up with the work in the weaving shed—had been admitted by the Elders to the program as a kind of compensation when Das resigned. Das was probably considered eligible for the same reason; that, and the fact that he could still do some useful work in the office. While other members of the scheme watered coconut palms which they then sat beneath for the remainder of their shift, Das could be used to prepare a budget or to answer a bundle of correspondence in the same time period, and he could even still be called upon to lead a delegation to see Mr. Klausman or another donor.

I was slightly surprised by the development though because Gurumurthy, his long time office rival, had finally won himself the job of project co-ordinator and could, had he wanted to have done so, blocked Das's inclusion—particularly as he still owed so much money to the office. Vishnu, an outsider who had been appointed after Das left, had lasted only a year, largely out of dissatisfaction with the salary and his pregnant wife's unhappiness about having to live in a provincial backwater where she knew no-one. Gurumurthy, when I asked him, told me it was out of genuine compassion for a former colleague down on his luck, but Das was probably right to be sceptical. "I think he thought I could be useful to him," Das speculated. "I could do the paperwork, calculate the budgets for the different programmes—things he found difficult."

Whatever the reasons behind it, at the end of the year he was called to the office and offered an extended role as quality checker in the weaving shed, a post that had been agreed by the Management Committee. It might have been Vibulananthan's influence, now serving on the committee, that swung it, but the logic was that it was better to have Das working for them, and some of his wages cut to pay off his debts, than have him outside and paying nothing. "There was no salary, no pension or anything like that," said Das, "but they told me they would pay me Rs96 per day, with Rs24 deducted for outstanding debts. This was late 2007, early 2008. I thought, why not? It's good to have some kind of income, and the burden is not so heavy, so I should be able to manage the work."

"A couple of months later, Gurumurthy asked if I could look after one of the new income generating schemes they were setting up. There was a donor who wanted to give out loans to older people and get them self-supporting, so we started with four people, one for a petty shop, one for land rearing, another one for buying and keeping chickens. So I did that and other things."

The scheme foundered soon after Das's initial work on it, not because of anything Das had done but because things were once again coming to a head in Anandapuram's office, and the project was lost in the fall out. Das must have been relived that, this time, it was not about him, but about his current successor, Gurumurthy. "I wasn't there in the office when it all happened," Das told me, "but you could hear the shouting going on from the weaving shed. Things had been building up for sometime. He was accused of taking money by using duplicate bills: overcharging for expenses and pocketing the rest."

"He had also been drinking more and more. Someone had told the Elders that he was using Anil, the young boy who was training to be a cobbler, to go out and bring him whisky to drink, so they trapped him one day, caught Anil on the way back from the bazaar and demanded to see what he's bought and who it was for. But everyone knew anyway: Gurumurthy was even drinking in the office—that's why, I think, he had a fridge in there, to keep the soda and ice in! Anyway, one day he'd had his full of drink and had gone home to sleep it off, leaving Baburao and the other staff to make the custodial care payment. He wasn't very well, by then, either. His legs were very swollen, whether because of the drink or something else I don't know. Anyway, they set up a table outside the weaving unit with the cash box and the books, and then everyone queued up for their money as usual, either to sign for it in the book or put a thumbprint there. But when they were doing it, Gurumurthy suddenly turned up, still drunk, and sat alongside the staff while they made the payments. He started being rude and shouting at the old people as they came for their money. One woman had come to collect her sister's payment because the sister was sick and couldn't come for it herself. He used vulgar words against her, told her that her sister would need to come for herself. 'Do you all know how hard I have to work to bring this money in for all of you!' he yelled at them. 'It's not your fathers' or your mothers' money! It's not from your own work! It's from me!' Then he turned to Baburao, who was sitting there next to him, and started on him. 'And what are you staring at?' he said, 'You want to do something against me, do you?!' It was all very ugly. Lots of the old people went off and made a complaint to the Elders, said this wasn't an acceptable way to do things. That was the start of it."

By the time I saw Das again in the summer of 2009—when I was interviewing him for this book—Gurumurthy had been pushed to resign, and a new project co-ordinator, Suresh, was in post. Das, it seemed, found himself a niche. "I might be in the weaving shed for three or four days, followed by another three or four days in the office and other places: that's how it seems to go. I don't do the quality checking any more: I make up the orders, calculate wages, do a bit of purchasing if that's what's called for. I'm not suitable for quality checking any more—my eyes are not good enough, not at my age. I just help out where I can." Das was officially on leave during much of my stay that year, spending his time talking to me on my verandah or travelling back to the places he had once lived so that we could retrace his story. Nevertheless, the interruptions we got demonstrated how much he was still involved in things.

"Das, you're wanted in the crèche!" Kotaiah, one of the office messengers, called from the end of the pathway to my house one morning, when we were in mid flow.

"We're at the climax of my life story!" he shouted back, laughing. "Tell them I'll come and look at the crèche accounts after lunch."

"Okay," replied Kotaiah, "I'll tell her. But soon the hero of the story will have to run away and do his work!"

Das seemed nearly as relaxed as he had done two years earlier, when I worked with him soon after the death of his mother. People in the village complained about Suresh as much as they had complained about Raj Kumar, Das included, but he no longer nursed ambitions of returning to the role of project co-ordinator, and when he complained of the current post holder's incompetence it was with less rancour than in the past. He still enjoyed gossiping about it, but he no longer cared so much what the upshot would be.

He no longer complained to me of crippling debts, either; and, given our history, I declined to ask. I was paying him for his time, and he appeared to be managing. The things that had marked his return to prosperity on my last visit were no longer there, however. The china cup with the daffodil on it was broken; Mariya's gold had been sold to pay off debts (without her throat being cut); and the inherited furniture had taken a battering. Mariya was friendly when I visited, but there were no repeated dinner invitations, and this time when I was offered tea it was sent for from the teashop. Her laughter at Das's jokes had been replaced by her more familiar scowls.

At least there was still the money held in trust for his children, so although neither of them were attending school any more there was at least some safety net in place for them. Joshua, he said, would in any case be all right. "He's clever even if he's not educated, so he'll be okay, I think. No-one took much care of me either, but I survived, and look at all the lives I've lived! I've married, worked, had children—despite a life on the stations and with leprosy. One day he'll understand what to do. If he's hungry he'll find a way to earn. God will help him in some way."

Joshua had started at the high school across the railway lines and initially seemed to have been doing well, but, like his sister, he was put off from attending. "After the half yearly exams there was a holiday, and he never went back again after that. The teacher used to beat him because his hands sweated so much . . . he couldn't help it, but his condition meant the ink ran in his exercise books, and they'd accuse him of spilling water on it. So that was that. He was afraid to go back, and now he spends his time wandering, playing cricket, doing whatever mischief he can . . . there are too many other boys not going to school for him to hang around with!"

He also—I heard from a disapproving villager, who thought a family of Das's status should be setting a better example—had been working. Das was happy to admit it. "Yes, I encouraged him!" he said, "If he wasn't going to school and wasn't interested in helping his mother, why not?" The fifteen-year-old daughter of one of their neighbours, Jansi, was already working in one of the new readymade clothing shops that had opened in the nearby town, and she had offered to take Joshua along with her. "She's very clever," Das told me. "She gets left there in charge by the shop owner, and she does a good job of getting money out of the customers. She'll stand there behind the counter, pulling down shirts and other things to show the customer. 'How much is that one?' they'll say, and she tells them: 'Oh, Rs780, that one sir. Good choice, top quality!' Actually, the thing she's showing them will only be worth Rs180! And the customer will think to himself, hmm, Rs780. That's a lot, but I can try to get a bargain, to haggle for Rs400. So he'll start by offering Rs350, and she'll say, 'No, no no! These are top quality garments sir. If you like, I can bring you out lower quality items.' And in the end she'll sell it to him for Rs500—so the shop owner, he's very pleased!"

"He couldn't do it himself—he'd get a bad reputation—but it's okay if his shop girl does it, and if there's any problem, if a customer starts making a fuss, he can come into the shop and intervene, explain that she's only young, was just minding the shop, that she made a mistake. He'll take over the transaction and sell at the proper price. But mostly he'll leave her to it— watching over the shop on CCTV—and will be in one of his other shops."

Joshua started working alongside her, six days a week, each day until the shop drew down its shutters at around 10:30pm, when he would cycle home. His job was to climb up the high shelves above Jansi's head, throwing down items for her to show customers and folding them up afterwards. "And at least he went along, and stayed there once he arrived, so he wasn't getting up to any mischief there, and I thought, well, if he sticks it out for a year or two maybe he'll learn the business and will be better placed to do something like that himself. That's why I left him there."

He earned Rs600—around half of Jansi's wage—but the owner, impressed by Jansi's sales techniques, turned a blind eye to her taking a cut of the extra she took on her transactions, and allowed them to take money from the till to buy themselves bhajis or jalabi, cups of tea and the occasional *badam palu* (almond milk), sweet and yellow with cashew nuts at the bottom. Joshua was even able to buy his family clothes at Christmas time: "I wore the shirt he gave me, that nice blue one I had on when we were in Kumbakonam!" Das said, proudly. "Of course, he got them on credit and left before he'd fully paid the shop owner back. When he sees Joshua in the town he calls out to him: 'Hey! Pay me what you owe or come back to work!' But Joshua can run faster than him! He stopped going there in February, around the time Jansi left and got married. He got lazy, or the shop keeper ordered him around and he didn't like it, so he lost interest. He's thirteen or fourteen, no? Boys want to run around and be free. But he was there for five months."

Das sighed and looked thoughtful for a moment. "People are always telling me—to my face, sometimes; sometimes behind my back—that I should have done more for my children's future. But how do we know what will happen, even tomorrow? What was written on their foreheads when they were born we don't know: if they need to suffer, they need to suffer. I saw a film once about two tribal girls who lived in a small hut and survived by selling pins and needles. One day, a Rs1,000 note fluttered toward them— more money than they had ever seen. It was an old film, so it really was a fortune. One of the girls caught it, and, to ensure it didn't get stolen, they put it in a tin and buried it somewhere in the house. But whereas previously they had been able to enjoy themselves freely, now they spent all their time worrying about whether someone might come and take their money. One of the girls fell ill and then, because she was lying there fretting about the safety of the money, she even failed to notice a venomous snake enter the hut. It bit her and she died. Then there was a flood, and water got into the box and spoiled the money anyway. There were some other sub-plots and a few comic routines in the film too, but this was the central story. So perhaps it is better not to think too much about the future, and to do what we can now."

"And with Kaveri, well, that money is there from my mother if we need to give any dowry, and after she's married her husband can take care of her. Joshua, like I said, will take care of himself. As for Mariya, well, if I die before she does, she has this little house, her custodial care money and her leprosy pension, so she'll manage if she needs to. But she's weak and anemic: she probably won't live much beyond fifty, so she might even go first!"

"As for me, I'm sixty now, so who knows? If I die in the next year or two maybe Mariya will remarry—I hope she does! But I wouldn't marry again. It's too late with Padma, I'm too old—my desire is spent!—and anyway she has her own husband. The time for that has passed. Maybe when I was forty-five, even fifty. But not now: Mariya is here, the two children are here, and I don't want to harm any of them. So no, I won't be running away!"

We stopped talking then: his life, no doubt, would continue in its twists and turns, but he had taken me up to the present. I turned off my tape recorder, we drank some tea, and I went off to the guesthouse to finish my packing. I was sad to be going; it was a relief to have finished the interviews before I had to leave, but there was also something poignant about having come to the end of the story. I had almost finished gathering my things together when there was a knock on the screen door, and I pulled it back, thinking the driver who was taking me to the station had arrived early.

It was Das's brother Chandra Prakash on the verandah, though, and he was beaming. "I told you my story the other day," he said, "and I wanted you to be able to write down a happy ending!" He beckoned me to the end of the path where, illuminated by the flickering street lamp, was a shiny new yellow auto rickshaw, the names of his two sons emblazoned across the front, loud speakers for projecting music or messages sprouting from the roof, and seats covered in a kitsch design of bananas, apples and oranges on a shiny blue background. "It's mine!" he said happily, explaining that he had bought the vehicle with a bank loan and would be using it to taxi people to and from the market or wherever else they wanted to go. It was already full of neighboring children—including Joshua and Kaveri, who were laughing noisily in the back—and he was going for a spin around the outer perimeter of the colony. At his request, I took a photograph. "Now you have an end for your book," he said, helpfully. Although this was ostensibly a story about his brother, Chandra Prakash clearly saw things differently. Conforming to the claims of those anthropologists who argue that Indians tend to experience themselves as continuous with others rather than as bounded, self-determining individuals—as "familial selves"—he appeared to be making no absolute distinction between Das's life and his own.[4] "In our family we've had lots of difficulties," he added. "But now I have this new three-wheeler, our children are all healthy, and I think everything is going to be all right!"

NOTES

1. There is a growing literature on India's so-called "emerging" middle classes. See, for example, I. Ahmad, and H. Reifeld (eds), *Middle Class Values in India and Western Europe* (New Delhi: Social Science Press, 2003); Minna, Säävälä, "Auspicious Hindu houses. The new middle classes in Hyderabad, India," *Social Anthropology* 11, 2 (2003): 231–247; Henrike Donner, and Geert De Neve, "Introduction," In *Being Middle-class in India: A Way of Life*, (Oxon: Routledge, 2003) pp1–22; L. Fernandes, *India's New Middle Class: Democratic Politics in an Era of Economic Reform* (Minneapolis: University of Minnesota, 2006).

2. For anthropological reflection on the tsunami and its aftermath more generally, see Rod Stirrat, "Competitive Humanitarianism: Relief and the Tsunami in Sri Lanka," *Anthropology Today*, 22, 5 (2006): 11–16.

3. In addition to Sitrrat, "Competitive Humanitarianism" on the tsunami in particular, for recent contributions to the anthropology of aid more generally, see David Mosse and David Lewis (eds.), *Development Brokers and Translators. The Ethnography of Aid and Agencies* (Bloomfield, CT: Kumarian Press, 2006); David Mosse (ed.), *Adventures in Aidland: The Anthropology of Professionals in International Development* (New York; Oxford: Berghahn Press, 2011); and David Mosse, *Cultivating Development: An Ethnography of Aid Policy and Practice* (London; Ann Arbor, MI.: Pluto Press, 2005).

4. See, for proponents of this argument, McKim Marriott, Constructing an Indian Ethnosociology. *Contributions to Indian Sociology* (N.S.) 23 (1989): 1–39; and, from a psychological perspective, Alan Roland, *In Search of the Self in India and Japan: Toward a Cross-Cultural Psychology*. New Jersey: Princeton University Press, 1988; Sudhir Kakar, *Culture and Psyche: Selected Essays*. Delhi: Oxford University Press, 1997. I also engage with critics of this position in Staples, "Disguise, Revelation and Copyright."

Bibliography

Ahmad, I. and H. Reifeld (eds), *Middle Class Values in India and Western* Europe. New Delhi: Social Science Press, 2003.

Alter, Joseph. *Knowing Dil Das: Stories of a Himalayan Hunter*. Philadelphia: University of Pennsylvania Press, 2000.

Arnold, David and Stuart Blackburn, 2004. "Introduction: Life Histories in India." In *Telling Lives in India: Biography, Autobiography and Life History*, edited by David Arnold and Stuart Blackburn (Bloomington: Indiana University Press, 2004) 1–28.

Awasthi, Shailendra. "From Matka king to anonymous punter, life's come a full circle for him," *Express India* (December 2, 2007), accessed May 29, 2013, http://expressindia. indianexpress.com/latest-news/From-Matka-king-to-anonymous-punter-lifes-come-a-full-circle-for-him/245717/

Barley, Nigel. *The Innocent Anthropologist: Notes from a Mud Hut*. Prospect Heights, Illinois: Waveland Press, 2000.

Bayly, Susan. *Caste, Society and Politics in India from the Eighteenth Century to the Modern Age*, Cambridge: Cambridge University Press, 1999.

Bean, Susan S. "Toward a Semiotics of 'Purity' and 'Pollution' in India." *American Ethnologist*, 8, 3 (1981): 575–595.

Beatty, Andrew. "How Did It Feel For You? Emotion, Narrative, and the Limits of Ethnography." *American Anthropologist*, 112, 3 (2010): 430–443.

Beatty, Andrew. *A Shadow Falls: In the Heart of Java*. London: Faber and Faber, 2009.

Beatty, Andrew. *Society and Exchange in Nias*. Oxford: Oxford University Press, 1992.

Beatty, Andrew. *Varieties of Javanese Religion: an Anthropological Account*. Cambridge: Cambridge University Press, 1999.

Bennett, Lynne. *Dangerous Wives and Sacred Sisters: Social and Symbolic Roles of High Caste Women in Nepal*. New York: Columbia University Press, 1983.

Béteille, Andre. *Caste, Class and Power: Changing Patterns of Social Stratification in a Tanjore Village*. Oxford: Oxford University Press, 1996.

Bourdieu, Pierre. *Outline of a Theory on Practice*. Cambridge: Cambridge University Press, 1972.

Brown, Carolyn Henning. "The Forced Sterilization Program Under the Indian Emergency: Results in One Settlement," *Human Organization*, 43, 1 (1984): 49–54.

Brown, Karen McCarthy. *Mama Lola: A Vodou Priestess in Brooklyn*. Berkeley: University of California Press, 1991.

Buckingham, Jane. *Leprosy in Colonial South India*. London: Palgrave, 2002.

Burnham, Michelle. "'I Lied All the Time': Trickster Discourse and Ethnographic Authority in 'Crashing Thunder.'" *American Indian Quarterly*, 22, 4 (1988): 469–484.

Busby, Cecilia. *The Performance of Gender: An Anthropology of Everyday Life in a South Indian Fishing Village*. New Brunswick: Althone Press, 2000.

Caplan, Pat. "The transcendent subject? Biography as a medium for writing 'life and times.'" In *Extraordinary Encounters: Authenticity and the Interview*, edited by Katherine Smith, James Staples and Nigel Rapport, Oxford: Berghahn, 2015.

Cassidy, Rebecca. *The Sport of Kings: Kinship, Class and Thoroughbred Breeding in Haymarket*. Cambridge: Cambridge University Press, 2002.

Chernoff, John. *Hustling is Not Stealing: Stories of an African Bar Girl*. Chicago: University of Chicago Press, 2003.

Clifford, James and George Marcus (eds.) *Writing Culture: The Poetics and Politics of Ethnography*. Berkeley: University of California Press, 1985.

Clifford, James. "On Ethnographic Authority," *Representations* 1, 2 (1983): 118–146.

Crapanzano, Vincent. *Tuhami: Portrait of a Moroccan* Chicago: University of Chicago Press, 1980.

de Bruin, M. H. *Leprosy in South India: Stigma and Strategies of Coping*. Pondy Paper in Social Sciences: Institute Francais de Pondicherry, 1996.

de Certeau, Michel. *The Practice of Everyday Life*. Berkeley: University of California Press, 1984.

Deliége, Robert. *The Untouchables of India*. Translated by Nora Scott. Oxford: Berg, 1999.

Desai, Amit and Evan Killick, eds., *The Ways of Friendship: Anthropological Perspectives*. Oxford: Berghahn, 2010.

Desjarlais, Robert. *Sensory Biographies: Lives and Deaths Among Nepal's Yolmo Buddhists*. Berkeley: University of California Press, 2003.

Dhar, P. N. *Indira Gandhi, the 'Emergency' and Indian Democracy*. New Delhi: Oxford University Press, 2000.

Dharmalingam, A. "The Social Context of Family Planning In a South Indian Village," *International Family Planning Perspectives*, 21, 3 (1995): 98–103.

Dogra, R. C. and U. Dogra, *Thought Provoking Hindu Names*, New Delhi: Star Publications, 2008.

Donner, Henrike, and Geert De Neve. "Introduction." In *Being Middle-class in India: A Way of Life*. Oxon: Routledge (2003) pp1–22.

Donner, Henrike. *Domestic Goddesses: Maternity, Globalization and Middle-class Identity in Contemporary India*. Farnham: Ashgate, 2008.

Dumont, Louis and David Pocock. "Pure and Impure." *Contributions to Indian Sociology* 3 (1959): 9–39.

Dumont, Louis. *Homo Hierarchicus, the Caste System and Its Implications*. Chicago and London: University of Chicago Press, 1980.

Edmond, Rod. *Leprosy and Empire: A Medical and Cultural History*. Cambridge: Cambridge University Press, 2006.

Evans-Pritchard, E. E. *The Nuer: A Description of the Models of Livelihood and Political Institutions of a Nilotic People*. Oxford: Oxford University Press, 1940.

Farmer, Paul. *Pathologies of Power: Health, Human Rights, and the New War on the Poor*. Berkeley: University of California Press, 2005.

Fernandes, L. *India's New Middle Class: Democratic Politics in an Era of Economic Reform*. Minneapolis: University of Minnesota, 2006.

Frank, Gelya. "Anthropology and individual lives: the story of the life history and the life history of the story," *American Anthropologist*, 97 (1995): 145–148.

Frank, Gelya. *Venus on Wheels: Two Decades of Dialogue on Disability, Biography and Being Female in America*. Berkeley: California University Press, 2000.

Frank, Katherine. *Indira: The Life of Indira Nehru Gandhi*. London: Harper Collins, 2010.

Freeman, James M. *Untouchable: an Indian Life History*. London: Allen and Unwin, 1979.

Froerer, Peggy. "Close Friends: The Importance of Proximity in the Formation of Friendship in Chhattisgarh, India." In *The Ways of Friendship: Anthropological Perspectives*, edited by Amit Desai and Evan Killick, 133–153.Oxford: Berghahn, 2010.

Fruzzetti, Lina M. *The Gift of a Virgin: Women, Marriage, and Ritual in a Bengali Society*. Delhi: Oxford University Press, 1990.

Fuller, C. J. "The modern transformation of an old elite: the case of the Tamil Brahmins." In *A Companion to the Anthropology of India*, edited by Isabelle Clark-Decès, 80–97. Chichester: Wiley-Blackwell, 2011.

Fuller, C. J. "Misconceiving the grain heap: a critique of the concept of the 'Indian jajmani system.'" In *Money and the Morality of Exchange*, edited by Jonathan Parry and Maurice Bloch, 33–36. Cambridge: Cambridge University Press, 1989.

Fuller, C. J. ed. *Caste Today*. Delhi: Oxford University Press, 1997.

Fuller, C. J. *The Camphor Flame: Popular Hinduism and Society in India*. Princeton: Princeton University Press, 2004.

Gardner, Katy and David Lewis. *Anthropology, Development and the Post-modern Challenge*. London: Pluto Press, 1996.

Geertz, Clifford. "Deep Play: Notes on the Balinese Cockfight." *Daedalus* 101, 1 (1972): 1–37.

Gorringe, Hugo and Irene Rafanell. "The Embodiment of Caste: Oppression, Protest and Change." *Sociology* 41, 1 (2007): 97–114.

Grindal, Bruce T. and Frank A. Salamone (eds.) *Bridges to Humanity: Narratives on Fieldwork and Friendship*. Long Grove, Illinois: Waveland Press, 2006.

Gupta, Dipankar. [ed.] *Caste in Question: Identity or Hierarchy?* New Delhi: Sage, 2004.

Gupta, Dipankar. *Interrogating Caste*. New Delhi: Penguin Books India, 2000.

Hacking, Ian. *Mad Travelers: Reflections on the Reality of Transient Mental Illnesses*. Cambridge, Mass: Harvard University Press, 1998.

Hardgrave, Robert L. Jr and Stanley A. Kochanek. *India: Government and Politics in a Developing Nation*. Boston: Thompson Wadsworth, 2008.

Henderson, Michael. *Experiment with Untruth: India under Emergency*. Delhi: Macmillan, 1977.

Ingold, Tim. *The Perception of the Environment: Essays in Livelihood, Dwelling and Skill*. London: Routledge, 2000.

Jeffery, Patricia. *Frogs in a Well. Indian Women in Purdah*. London: Zed Press, 1979.

Jeffrey, Craig. "Timepass: Youth, Class, and Time Among Unemployed Young Men in India." *American Ethnologist*, 7, 3 (2010a): 465–481.

Jeffrey, Craig. *Timepass: Youth, Class, and the Politics of Waiting in India*. Stanford: Stanford University Press, 2010b.

Jenkins, Richard. *Pierre Bourdieu*. London: Routledge, 1992.

Kakar, Sudhir, *Culture and Psyche: Selected Essays*. Delhi: Oxford University Press, 1997.

Knott, Kim. *Hinduism: A Very Short Introduction*. Oxford: Oxford University Press, 1998.

Krupat, Arnold. *For Those Who Came After: A Study of Native American Autobiography*. Berkeley: University of California Press, 1985.

Lamb, Sarah. *White Saris and Sweet Mangoes: Aging, Gender, and Body in North India*. Berkeley: University of California Press, 2000.

Langness, L.L. and Gelya Frank. *Lives: An Anthropological Approach to Biography*. Novato, California: Chandler and Sharp Publishers, Inc. 1981.

Lassiter, Luke Eric. *The Chicago Guide to Collaborative Ethnography*. Chicago: Chicago University Press, 2005.

Leach, Melissa and James Fairhead. *Vaccine Anxieties: Global Science, Child Health & Society*. London: Earthscan, 2007.

Lévi-Strauss, Claude. *Tristes Tropiques*, English translation by John and Doreen Weightman, New York: Atheneum, 1973.

Linde, Charlotte. *Life Stories: The Creation of Coherence*. New York: Oxford University Press, 1993.

Mageo, Jeannette Marie "Figurative Dream Analysis and U.S. Traveling Identities," *Ethnos* 34, 4 (2006): 456–487.

Malinowski, Bronislaw. Argonauts of the Western Pacific: An Account of Native Enterprise and Adventure in the Archipelagoes of Melanesian New Guinea. London: Routledge and Kegan Paul, 1922.

Marcus, George E. and Michael M. J. Fischer (eds.) *Anthropology as Cultural Critique: An Experimental Moment in the Human Sciences*. Chicago: University of Chicago Press, 1986.

Marglin, Frederique Apfell. "Power, Purity and Pollution: Aspects of the Caste System Reconsidered." *Contributions to Indian Sociology* (NS) 11, 2 (1977): 245–270.

Marriott, McKim and Ronald Inden. "Toward an Ethnosociology of South Asian Caste Systems." In *The New Wind: Changing Identities in South Asia*, edited by K. David. The Hague: Mouton, 1977, 227–238.

Marriott, McKim, "Constructing an Indian Ethnosociology." *Contributions to Indian Sociology* (N.S.) 23 (1989): 1–39.

Marriott, McKim. "Caste ranking and food transactions: A matrix analysis." In *Structure and Change in Indian Society*, edited by M. Singer, and B. S. Cohn, 133–71. Chicago: Aldine, 1968.

Mayer, Adrian. *Caste and Kinship in Central India: A Village and Its Region*. London: Routledge, 1960.

Mayer, Peter. "Inventing village tradition: the late nineteenth century origins of the north Indian 'jajmani system.'" *Modern Asian Studies* 27 (1993) 357–395.

McGuire, Meredith Lindsay. " 'How to sit, how to stand': bodily praxis and the new urban middle class." In *A Companion to the Anthropology of India*, edited by Isabelle Clark-Decès, 117–136. Wiley-Blackwell: Oxford, 2011.

McIntosh, Ian and Angus Erskine. " 'Money for nothing'? Understanding giving to beggars." *Sociological Research Online* 5, 1, 2000. http://www.socresonline.org.uk/5/1/mcintosh. html .

Menon, Nivedita. [ed.] *Gender and Politics in India*. Oxford: Oxford University Press, 1999.

Mintz, Sidney W. *Worker in the Cane: A Puerto Rican Life History*. New Haven: Yale University Press, 1960.

Mistry, Rohinton. *A Fine Balance*. London: Faber and Faber, 1996.

Moffatt, Michael. *An Untouchable Community in South India: Structure and Consensus*. Princeton, N.J.: Princeton University Press, 1979.

Moon, Vasant. *Growing Up Untouchable in India: a Dalit Autobiography*. Landham, Maryland: Rowman and Littlefield, 2001.

Mosse, David and Lewis, David (eds.) *Development Brokers and Translators. The Ethnography of Aid and Agencies*. Bloomfield, CT: Kumarian Press, 2006.

Mosse, David, (ed.) *Adventures in Aidland: The Anthropology of Professionals in International Development*. New York; Oxford: Berghahn Press, 2011.

Mosse, David, *Cultivating Development: An Ethnography of Aid Policy and Practice*. London; Ann Arbor, MI.: Pluto Press, 2005.

Narayan, Kirin. *Alive in the Writing: Crafting Ethnography in the Company Of Chekhov*. Chicago: Chicago University Press, 2012.

Narayan, Kirin. *Love, Stars and all That*. New York: Pocket Books, 1994.

Narayan, Kirin. *My Family and Other Saints*. Chicago: University of Chicago Press, 2007.

Navon, L. "Beggars, metaphors and stigma." *Social History of Medicine*, 11(1998): 89–105.

Niehaus, Isak. *Witchcraft and a Life in the New South Africa*. Cambridge: Cambridge University Press, 2012.

Niehaus, Isak. *Witchcraft, Power and Politics: Exploring the Occult in the South African Lowveld*. London: Pluto Press, 2001.

Oddie, Geoffrey. *Hindu and Christian in South-East India*. London: Curzon Press, 1991.

Panandiker, Pai. *Family Planning under the Emergency: Policy Implications and Incentives and Disincentives* (New Delhi: Radiant Publishers, 1978.

Parry, Jonathan. "The Koli Dilemma." *Contributions to Indian Sociology* (N.S.) 4 (1970): 84–104.

Parry, Jonathan. "The marital history of 'A Thumb-Impression man.'" In *Telling Lives in India: Biography, Autobiography and Life History*, edited by David Arnold and Stuart Blackburn, 281–318. Bloomington: Indiana University Press, 2004.

Peacock, James L. and Dorothy C. Holland. "The Narrated Self: Life Stories in Process." *Ethos* 21, 4 (1993): 367–383.

Pettigrew, Joyce. "Take Not Arms Against Thy Sovereign: The Present Punjab Crisis and the Storming of the Golden Temple." *South Asia Research* 4, 2 (1984):102.

Pottier, Johan. [ed.] *Practising Development: Social Science Perspectives*. London: Routledge, 1993.
Price, John A. "Gambling in Traditional Asia." *Anthropologica* (NS) 14, 2 (1972): 157–180.
Racine, Josiane and Jean-Luc Racine. "Beyond Silence: A Dalit Life History in South India." In *Telling Lives in India: Biography, Autobiography and Life History*, edited by David Arnold and Stuart Blackburn, 252–280 (Bloomington: Indiana University Press, 2004).
Radhakrishnan, Smitha. *Appropriately Indian: Gender and Culture in a New Transnational Class*. Durham, NC: Duke University Press, 2011.
Radin, Paul. *Crashing Thunder: The Autobiography of an American Indian*. Michigan: Michigan University Press, 1999.
Roland, A. *In Search of the Self in India and Japan: Toward a Cross-Cultural Psychology*. New Jersey: Princeton University Press, 1988.
Rosenwald, George C. & Richard L. Ochberg. 1992. *Storied Lives: The Cultural Politics of Self-Understanding*. New Haven: Yale University Press.
Rushdie, Salman. *Midnight's Children*. London: Penguin, 1991.
Säävälä, Minna, "Auspicious Hindu houses. The new middle classes in Hyderabad, India." *Social Anthropology* 11, 2 (2003): 231–247.
Sanjek, Roger. "Anthropology's hidden colonialism: assistants and their ethnographers." *Anthropology Today* 9, 2 (April 1993): 13–18.
Sarin, Ritu. *The Assassination of Indira Gandhi*, New Delhi: Penguin Books, 1990.
Searle-Chattterjee, Mary and Ursula Sharma. [eds.,] *Contextualising Caste*. Oxford: Blackwell, 2004.
Sharma, Kalpana. *Rediscovering Dharavi: Stories from Asia's largest slum*. New Delhi: Penguin India, 2000.
Silla, Eric. *People Are Not the Same: Leprosy and Identity in Twentieth-Century Mali*. Oxford: James Currey, 1998.
Simmons, Leo W. (ed.) *Sun Chief: The Autobiography of a Hopi Indian*. New Haven: Yale University Press, 1942.
Singh, Gurharpal. "Understanding the 'Punjab Problem.'" *Asian Survey* 27, 12 (1987): 1268–1277.
Smith, Mary. *Baba of Karo: A Woman of the Muslim Hausa*. New Haven: Yale University Press. 1981.
Spencer, Jonathan. *A Sinhala Village in a Time of Trouble: Politics and Change in Rural Sri Lanka*. New Delhi: Oxford University Press, 2000.
Srinivas, M. N. (ed.) *Caste: Its Twentieth Century Avatar*. New Delhi: Penguin Books India, 1997.
Staples, James and Katherine Smith. "Introduction." in *Extraordinary Encounters: Authenticity and the Interview*, edited by Katherine Smith, James Staples and Nigel Rapport. Oxford: Berghahn, 2015.
Staples, James and Tom Widger. "Situating Suicide as an Anthropological Problem: Ethnographic Approaches to Understanding Self-Harm and Self-Inflicted Death," *Culture, Medicine and Psychiatry* 36, 2 (2012) 183–203.
Staples, James. "'Go on, just try some!': Meat and Meaning-Making among South Indian Christians." *South Asia: Journal of South Asian Studies* (NS) 31, 1 (2008):36–55.
Staples, James. "An 'up and down life': understanding leprosy through biography." In *Extraordinary Encounters: The ethnographic interview, biography and authentic data*, edited by Katherine Smith, James Staples and Nigel Rapport (Oxford: Berghahn, forthcoming).
Staples, James. "Becoming a man: Personhood and masculinity in a south Indian leprosy colony." *Contributions to Indian Sociology* 39, 2 (2005): 279–305.
Staples, James. "Culture and Carelessness: constituting disability in South India," *Medical Anthropology Quarterly* 26, 4 (2012): 557–74.
Staples, James. "Delineating disease: Self-management of leprosy identities in South India." *Medical Anthropology* 23, 1 (2004): 69–88.
Staples, James. "Disguise, Revelation and Copyright: Disassembling the South Indian Leper." *Journal of the Royal Anthropological Institute* (N.S.) 9 (2003): 295–315.

Staples, James. "Ethnographies of Suicide in South Asia." In *Suicide in South Asia: Ethnographic Perspectives*, ed. James Staples. Special Issue of *Contributions to Indian Sociology* 46, 1–2 (2012): 1–28.

Staples, James. "Leprosy and Alms collecting in Mumbai." In *Livelihoods at the Margins*, edited by James Staples, 163–186. Walnut Creek, California: Left Coast Press, 2007.

Staples, James. "Nuancing 'leprosy stigma' through ethnographic biography in South India," *Leprosy Review* 82, 2 (2011): 109–23.

Staples, James. "Putting Indian Christianities into context: biographies of Christian conversion in a leprosy colony." *Modern Asian Studies*. (2014, online).

Staples, James. "The suicide niche: accounting for self-harm in a South Indian leprosy colony," In *Suicide in South Asia: Ethnographic Perspectives*, ed. James Staples. Special Issue of *Contributions to Indian Sociology* 46, 1–2 (2012): 117–144.

Staples, James. "When things are not as they seem: Untangling the webs that hold together a South Indian NGO." In *Negotiating Boundaries and Borders: Qualitative Methodology and Development Research*, edited by Matt Smith, 131–154. Oxford: Elsevier, 2007.

Staples, James. *Peculiar People, Amazing Lives: Leprosy, Social Exclusion and Community Making in South India.* New Delhi: Orient Longman, 2007.

Stirrat, Rod. "Competitive Humanitarianism: Relief and the Tsunami in Sri Lanka," *Anthropology Today*, 22, 5 (2006): 11–16.

Stone, Linda and Caroline James. "Dowry, Bride-Burning, and Female Power in India." *Women's Studies International Forum* 18, 2 (1995): 125–43.

Swarup, Vikas. *Q & A.* London: Black Swan, 2006.

Tarlo, Emma. *Unsettling Memories: Narratives of the Emergency in India.* Berkeley: University of California Press, 2003.

Toofan, Brij Mohan. *When Freedom Bleeds: Journey through Indian Emergency.* Delhi: Ajanta Publications, 1988.

Van Maanen, John. *Tales of the Field: On Writing Ethnography.* Chicago: University of Chicago Press, 1988.

Viramma, Josiane Racine and Jean-Luc Racine. *Viramma: Life of an Untouchable.* Translated by Will Hobson. London: Verso, 1997.

Volpp, Leti. "Blaming culture for bad behaviour." *Yale Journal of Law and the Humanities* 12 (2000): 89–117.

White, Cassandra. *An Uncertain Cure: Living with Leprosy in Rio de Janeiro.* New Brunswick, New Jersey: Rutgers University Press, 2009.

Index

absconding, 5, 12, 17–18, 20, 23n3, 31, 52, 56, 60, 89
agency: lack of, 50, 117
alcohol: alcoholism, 73; arrack, 28; as prop, 116, 127; at festivals, 112; at work, 155; consumption of, 101, 106–107, 115; demands for, 127; drunkenness, 155–156; kallu (toddy), 115; Mariya's drinking of, 115; at work, 155. *See also* intoxicants
Andhra Pradesh: Hyderabad, 135, 135–136; Khammam, 72, 73; Nellore, 63; Vijayawada, 120
arguments: domestic, 90–91, 116; between anthropologist and research assistant, 144–145. *See also* violence

Bangalore, 57
Barara, 20
begging, 66–67, 73, 139; NGOs, reactions to, 122–123; *zanda* groups, 70, 71, 122–123. *See also* charity; gifting
Bible, book of Job, xiv. *See also* Christianity
biography, xvii. *See also* life history; research methods
Bombay, xiv, xv, xvi, 25; Bandara, 33; Bycula station, 39; Chembur, 27, 59; Colaba, xv; Dadar station, 32; Dharavi, 37; Goregaon, 26; Grant Road, 28; Juhu beach, 28; Mahalaxmi, 104; Santa Cruz,

26, 27; Tilak bridge, 33
Brahmins, xiii, 2, 62; behaviors of, 6, 77; discriminating, 121; food of, 7, 82, 154; Iyers, 2; pride in being, 140; relations between, 117; sex, 38; skin color, 22; speech, 46; style of drinking coffee, 3; vegetarianism, 36
bribery, 25, 33; in prison, 39; race fixing, 45, 52, 53, 103
buildings, 88; houses, 2, 65
bureaucracy, xiv

Calcutta, 20–21
caste: casteism, 121; conversion, and, 92; discrimination by, 2, 27; embodiment of, xviii, 7, 131; food rules, 7; identity, 38; Iyers. *See* Brahmins; low caste, 22, 51, 86; Madiga, 46, 72, 82, 90, 121, 131; Mala, 46, 90; Reddys, 90; scheduled castes and tribes, 15, 123; untouchables, xiii, xvi, xxv; Vaisyas, 2. *See also* Brahmins
charity, xix. *See also* begging
Chennai. *See* Madras
children and childhood, 1, 131, 132, 157; child labor, 157–158
Christianity: baptism, 74; calling to, 69; caste, in relation to, 123; Catholic church, 63, 138; meditation, 69; missionary organizations, 122; practices of, 75; prayer, 125, 126;

167

About the Author

JAMES STAPLES, PhD, is a senior lecturer in anthropology at Brunel University, London. He is author of *Peculiar People, Amazing Lives*, editor of *Livelihoods at the Margins,* and two recent volumes on suicide. He has also published numerous journal articles and chapters on his research in India.

Lightning Source UK Ltd.
Milton Keynes UK
UKOW05n1332170614

233593UK00001B/23/P

9 780739 187340